Pediatric Disorders

To the children and families who persevere and thrive despite battling the medical conditions described in this volume.

And to our families.

P.C.M. & S.R.S.

Pediatric Disorders

Paul C. McCabe
Steven R. Shaw

Current
Topics
and
Interventions
for
Educators

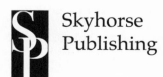
Skyhorse
Publishing

Skyhorse Publishing books may be purchased in bulk at special discounts for sales promotion, corporate gifts, fund-raising, or educational purposes. Special editions can also be created to specifications. For details, contact the Special Sales Department, Skyhorse Publishing, 307 West 36th Street, 11th Floor, New York, NY 10018 or info@skyhorsepublishing.com.

Skyhorse® and Skyhorse Publishing® are registered trademarks of Skyhorse Publishing, Inc.®, a Delaware corporation.

Visit our website at www.skyhorsepublishing.com.

10 9 8 7 6 5 4 3 2 1

Library of Congress Cataloging-in-Publication Data is available on file.

Cover design by Rose Storey

Print ISBN: 978-1-63220-561-2
Ebook ISBN: 978-1-63220-977-1

Printed in the United States of America

Contents

SECTION II: Current Issues in Pediatric Disorders and Treatments

Preface

This book exists for two primary reasons: (1) the incredible pressures on educators to address children's medical issues in school settings and (2) the rapid pace of news and information delivery, which often occurs despite safeguards that try to ensure credibility and verifiability. Educators are charged with making policies; differentiating instruction; providing educational accommodations; managing the physical plant; providing special education services; collaborating with families; and working with the community in response to children's medical, physical, and psychological issues. However, educators often have little training, support, or information to address these important issues. When faced with a medical question, many people (including us) turn to the Internet. Although much information from the Internet is of high quality, much is not. Peer-reviewed scientific papers of high quality are often given the same weight in search engine results as advertisements for the latest snake oil. Information about medical issues is presented in (1) esoteric medical science journals with little relevance to schooling, (2) an encyclopedic but cursory overview of many topics, or (3) simplified summaries on Web sites with questionable accuracy and oversight. We developed this book to give support and information to educators based on a critical review of scientific research that is credible, in depth, and practical.

Pediatric Disorders is the first book in a three-volume series entitled Current Topics and Interventions for Educators. This series presents detailed reviews of recent scientific research on a variety of topics in pediatrics that are most relevant to schools today. Current Topics and Interventions for Educators is intended to provide not only detailed scientific information on pediatric issues but also glossaries of key medical terms, educational strategies, case studies, handouts for teachers and parents, and discussion questions. Readers are presented with critical reviews of scientific medical research, including discussions of controversial issues. The authors of each chapter have completed scholarly reviews of the extant research and carefully considered the quality of research design, methodology, and sampling in determining what can be considered empirically valid conclusions versus conclusions based on opinion, conjecture, or myth. We believe that this information will help educators address the pediatric issues that affect schoolchildren and better equip educators to discuss these issues with parents, staff, and medical teams.

This book has its origins in a regular feature in the National Association of School Psychologists (NASP) publication *Communiqué* called "Pediatric School Psychology." We edited and published many detailed research articles that provided depth of information and critical evaluation of research to keep school psychologists current on medical knowledge that could impact their practice in the schools. We found that school psychologists shared this information with policy makers, administrators, social workers, teachers, therapists, and families. This feedback told us that there is wider audience for this information.

Educators, students, school nurses, administrators, policy makers, and school psychologists can use this book in a variety of ways. It can serve as a reference tool, textbook for a course, or a basis for continuing education activities in schools. The literature reviews are critical, challenge popular understanding, and often present controversial information. Therefore, we would also like the information in this book to serve as grist for discussion and debate. More than ever, educators are charged by law, regulation or circumstance to address medical issues despite lacking medical training. Therefore, consultation, reasoned discussion, debate, and consensus building can lead to improved educational services for children with medical and psychiatric issues.

Pediatric Disorders is a 13-chapter volume divided into three sections: (1) an introduction to schools as partners in health care delivery, (2) current medical issues affecting schoolchildren, and (3) prevention and wellness intervention in school settings. Schools are increasingly being asked to participate in health care delivery and oversight, and educators find themselves participating in collaborative problem-solving teams for students' health issues. Section II on current medical issues affecting schoolchildren covers the medical issues that receive the most media coverage, affect the most children, and generate the questions that educators most often hear. These pediatric disorders and their treatments include otitis media, childhood immunizations, shaken baby syndrome, sleep disorders, leukemia treatments, HIV, bacterial meningitis, and Lyme disease. Section III on prevention and wellness includes topics like obesity prevention, bullying prevention, and accident prevention. Although not inclusive, this volume covers topics that are among the most urgent and current in pediatrics in the schools.

—Paul C. McCabe and Steven R. Shaw, Editors

Acknowledgments

A large-scale project like this cannot take place without the assistance of many people. Jennifer Bruce and Sarita Gober provided many hours of editorial assistance in this project. Their support, skill, and good humor made this project possible. In addition, external reviewers read chapters and provided valuable comments. All chapters were improved because of the efforts of these students, educators, and scholars. The reviewers are Tiffany Chiu, Ray Christner, Jason Collins, Janine Fisher, Sarah Glaser, Sarita Gober, Terry Goldman, Michelle Harvie, Tom Huberty, Susan Jones, Robin Martin, Tawnya Meadows, Tia Ouimet, Mark Posey, Sara Quirke, Amira Rahman, Shohreh Rezazadeh, Jennifer Saracino, Christopher Scharf, Khing Sulin, and Jessica Carfolite Williams. Of course, the authors deserve the lion's share of appreciation, because their expertise, hard work, talent, and timeliness made this work possible. Many thanks for their expertise and generosity.

Paul McCabe would like to thank his colleagues at Brooklyn College of the City University of New York for their logistical support and encouragement of this project. He would also like to thank the many talented, hard-working graduate students who have worked with him over the years to contribute to the "Pediatric School Psychology" column and this project. Finally, he would like to offer grateful thanks to friends and family for their love and encouragement, especially to Dan.

Steven Shaw would like to thank the physicians from the Greenville Hospital System, South Carolina, who shaped his views of how education and pediatrics interact. Most notable of these physicians are Desmond Kelly, Nancy Powers, Mark Clayton, Lynn Hornsby, Curtis Rogers, James Beard, and William Schmidt. And, of course, thanks to Isabel, Zoe, and Joyce for their love, support, and patience.

About the Editors

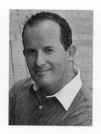

Paul C. McCabe, PhD, NCSP, is an Associate Professor of School Psychology in the School Psychologist Graduate Program at Brooklyn College of the City University of New York. Dr. McCabe received his PhD in Clinical and School Psychology from Hofstra University. He holds undergraduate degrees from University of Rochester and Cazenovia College. Dr. McCabe is a New York State-certified school psychologist, New York State-licensed psychologist, and a Nationally Certified School Psychologist (NCSP). Dr. McCabe serves on the editorial boards of several publications in school psychology and developmental psychology and has consulted at state and national levels on issues of early childhood assessment and best practices, pediatric issues in schools, and training in school psychology. Dr. McCabe conducts and publishes research in (1) early childhood social, behavioral, and language development and concomitant problems; (2) pediatric school psychology and health issues addressed by schools; and (3) social justice issues in training, especially training educators to advocate for gay, lesbian, bisexual, and transgendered youth.

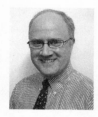

Steven R. Shaw, PhD, NCSP, is an Assistant Professor in the Department of Educational and Counselling Psychology at McGill University in Montreal, Quebec. Dr. Shaw received his PhD in School Psychology from the University of Florida. He has been a school psychologist since 1988 with clinical and administrative experience in schools, hospitals, and independent practice. He is editor-elect of *School Psychology Forum* and serves on the editorial board of several professional journals. He has conducted workshops and consulted with educational policy makers to address the needs of children with borderline intellectual functioning in the United States, Canada, Pakistan, Moldova, Poland, India, and Egypt. Dr. Shaw conducts and publishes research in (1) the development of children with rare genetic disorders; (2) resilience factors for children with risk factors for school failure, especially borderline intellectual functioning; and (3) pediatric school psychology and health issues addressed by schools.

About the Contributors

Laura Anderson, PhD, is Assistant Professor of Psychology at East Carolina University. She received her doctorate from the State University of New York at Buffalo. Her research interests include (1) prevention of health-related disorders, including childhood obesity; (2) ecological interventions for healthy weight promotion; (3) health disparities in diverse populations; (4) schoolwide positive behavior interventions and health promotion; and (5) program evaluation, particularly the efficacy of early literacy programs.

MaryBeth Bailar-Heath, MS, is a fourth-year graduate student in the clinical psychology doctoral program at Nova Southeastern University in Fort Lauderdale, Florida. Her primary clinical interests are in neuropsychology and rehabilitation psychology and more specifically in serving individuals with acquired brain injury. Bailar-Heath recently worked with her faculty mentors to implement an interdisciplinary rehabilitation program through Nova Southeastern for individuals who have sustained a traumatic brain injury. Bailar-Heath is also actively involved in leadership roles within the American Psychological Association of Graduate Students (APAGS).

Sarah A. Bassin, PhD, is a pediatric school psychologist with the University of South Carolina Medical School and school psychologist at Richland School District Two. Her clinical and research interests involve autism, developmental disabilities, and adjustment of children with medical issues.

Michelle Klein Brenner, MSEd, is a New York State–certified school psychologist and works as a school psychologist for the New York City Department of Education. She completed her graduate degree at Brooklyn College of the City University of New York and her undergraduate education at Yeshiva University, Stern College for Women. Ms. Brenner has previous publications for the National Association of School Psychologists, including an article in *Communiqué* and parent handouts. She is currently a doctoral candidate at the Graduate Center of the City University of New York. Ms. Brenner's research interests include cultural differences in cognitive, social, and emotional development; family systems; internalizing disorders of female adolescents; and ethics in professional practice.

Joseph A. Buckhalt, PhD, NCSP, is a Wayne T. Smith Distinguished Professor and the Director of the School Psychology Program at Auburn University. Dr. Buckhalt received his PhD from George Peabody College for Teachers, Vanderbilt University, and holds Licensure and National Certification in School Psychology. His research and scholarship have been related to assessment and treatment of children at risk for academic under-achievement and poor emotional/behavioral adjustment. Most recently, his work has been in collaboration with Dr. Mona El-Sheikh in studying how individual differences in sleep are related to educational and health outcomes in children.

Mona El-Sheikh, PhD, is Alumni Professor of Human Development and Family Studies at Auburn University, Alabama. She received her PhD from West Virginia University. Dr. El-Sheikh has been Principal Investigator on numerous research grants from the National Institutes of Health and the National Science Foundation and is the recipient of The Creative Scholarship Award from Auburn University. Her research has addressed biobehavioral mechanisms in children affected by stressors. Further, her integration of paradigms across scholarly disciplines and across different psychophysiological systems has resulted in better understanding of emotional, immune, and sleep regulation in children.

Sarah Glaser, BA, is a graduate student within the School/Applied Child Psychology Program at McGill University in Montreal, Quebec. She holds an undergraduate degree from Boston University. Ms. Glaser conducts research on the interaction between intellectual disabilities and mental health issues.

Rebecca Lakin Gullan, PhD, is a Research Fellow in the Community Schools Program in the Department of Psychology at The Children's Hospital of Philadelphia. Dr. Gullan earned her PhD in Clinical Psychology at Bowling Green State University, Ohio, with a specialization in children and families. Dr. Gullan is currently the Principal Investigator of a grant from the NICHD/NIH (Kirschstein National Research Service Award for Individual Postdoctoral Fellows) to develop a community service program to promote civic and ethnic identity in African American, urban youth. Dr. Gullan also serves on the Editorial Advisory Board of *School Psychology Quarterly* and is an ad hoc reviewer for several additional journals. Dr. Gullan's primary areas of research are (1) using partnership-based research methodology to develop culturally responsive interventions and measurement tools and (2) understanding, measuring, and promoting empowerment in disenfranchised populations.

Ron Hamlen, PhD, received his PhD in Plant Pathology and Nematology and postdoctoral training in Insect Pathology and Microbial Insect Control from the Pennsylvania State University. Dr. Hamlen also received a certificate in Health Risk Assessment from the Harvard School of Public Health. Dr. Hamlen is currently Vice President and Science Advisor for the Lyme Disease Association of Southeastern Pennsylvania and a member of the International Lyme and Associated Diseases Society, and he has served as a member of the Delaware Task Force to Examine the Prevalence of Lyme Disease in Delaware. Formerly a Biology Research Fellow and Global Technical Product Manager for E. I. DuPont de Nemours and Co., Inc. and an Associate Professor of Entomology and Nematology with the University of Florida, Dr. Hamlen, now retired, conducts public and corporate workshops and training forums for state government employees on Lyme disease and related tick-borne infections. Dr. Hamlen has published research and several review articles on Lyme disease, related tick-borne infections, and their prevention.

Jessica A. Hoffman, PhD, NCSP, is an Associate Professor in the Department of Counseling and Applied Educational Psychology at Northeastern University, Boston. Dr. Hoffman received her PhD in School Psychology at Lehigh University and completed her predoctoral internship and postdoctoral fellowship in pediatric psychology at the Children's Hospital of Philadelphia. Dr. Hoffman is a Massachusetts-licensed psychologist and school psychologist and holds the national certification in school psychology. She is the recipient of an early career (K) award from the National Institute of Child Health and Human Development to promote healthy eating in schools. Dr. Hoffman is on the editorial board of *School Psychology Review*. Her research focuses on the development of healthy eating behaviors among preschool and school-aged children.

Deborah S. Kliman, EdD, received her EdD from the University of Pennsylvania. Dr. Kliman also completed a postdoctoral fellowship in Structural Family Therapy at the Philadelphia Child Guidance Clinic. Dr. Kliman has had additional training in various types of psychotherapy, assessment, a variety of psychological disorders, and Lyme disease. Dr. Kliman's professional career has included preschool and first-grade teaching, directing a Head Start program, being a demonstration teacher at Trenton State College, and consulting in various areas of education and psychology, including 18 years at a battered women's shelter. Dr. Kliman was a professor of Child Development for 12 years at the University of Delaware and was a staff psychologist at a nonprofit clinic for families, children, and youth. Following her college teaching position, Dr. Kliman had a private practice in clinical psychology for more than 25 years and was licensed in Pennsylvania and Delaware. In the later years of her private practice, Dr. Kliman worked with many children and young people who were suffering from Lyme disease.

Fallon Lattari, MSEd, is a graduate of the School Psychologist Graduate Program at Brooklyn College of the City University of New York. She holds an undergraduate degree from Fordham University. Her research interests include early childhood issues, including food allergies and concomitant problems.

Tiffany Folmer Lawrence, MS, is a School Psychologist in the Avon Central High School, New York. She is a New York State–certified school psychologist. Ms. Lawrence received her MS and CAS in School Psychology from the Rochester Institute of Technology. She holds an undergraduate degree from Lafayette College. Professionally, Ms. Lawrence has an interest in response to intervention with secondary students, restorative justice practices in discipline, and Life Space Crisis Intervention.

Stephen S. Leff, PhD, is an Associate Professor of Clinical Psychology in the Department of Pediatrics at The Children's Hospital of Philadelphia and University of Pennsylvania School of Medicine. Dr. Leff received his PhD in Clinical Psychology from the University of North Carolina. He has been the Principal Investigator of four NIH-funded grants, all of which have been related to the use of partnership-based methods in the development, implementation, and evaluation of aggression prevention programs and assessment tools in the urban schools. He is currently conducting a clinical trial comparing a school-based relational aggression intervention (The Friend to Friend Program) to an educationally based intervention for urban, African American aggressive girls. Dr. Leff is also a Co-Investigator for the CDC-funded Philadelphia Collaborative Violence Prevention Center (PCVPC). Dr. Leff is on the Editorial Advisory Board for *School Psychology Review* and serves as an ad hoc reviewer for a number of additional journals, serves on two NIH Review Panels, and is involved in both regional and national groups related to bullying and victimization prevention. His research interests include school-based aggression prevention; social, cognitive, and gender differences in the expression of aggression; and partnership-based methods for intervention development.

Tia Ouimet is a graduate student in School/Applied Child Psychology in the Department of Educational and Counselling Psychology at McGill University in Montreal, Quebec. She received a BSc from McGill University in 2007 and was a research assistant in the McGill Child Development Laboratory for Research and Education in Developmental Disorders and the Resilience, Pediatric Psychology, and Neurogenetics Connections Laboratory before beginning her master's work with Dr. Steven Shaw in the Resilience, Pediatric Psychology, and Neurogenetics Connections Lab. Her research experience, as well as her clinical experience of working closely with children with autism, has led her to pursue research that has the goal of improving theory, assessment, and intervention implementation for children with developmental disorders.

Julie Paquette MacEvoy, PhD, is a Postdoctoral Fellow in the Department of Psychology at The Children's Hospital of Philadelphia. Dr. MacEvoy earned her PhD in clinical psychology from Duke University and earned a certificate degree in Developmental Psychology through a joint program between the University of North Carolina at Chapel Hill and Duke University. Dr. MacEvoy conducts and publishes research in (1) children's emotional experiences of their peer relationships, (2) the processes that are involved in the formation and maintenance of children's friendships, and (3) gender differences in children's anger and aggression toward peers.

W. Mark Posey, PhD, NCSP, is a School Psychologist and Codirector of the Department of Developmental Pediatrics at the University of South Carolina School of Medicine. He completed his doctoral degree at the University of South Carolina in School Psychology. Dr. Posey is licensed as a school psychologist in the state of South Carolina. His clinical and research interests include management of children with ADHD, the psychological adjustment of children with medical issues, and the assessment of children with autism.

Emily E. Powell, MA, is a psychology intern in the Department of Developmental Pediatrics at the University of South Carolina School of Medicine. Her research interests include autism and issues in intellectual disabilities.

Amy Racanello, MSEd, received her graduate degree from the School Psychologist Graduate Program of Brooklyn College of the City University in New York. She completed her undergraduate education at Cornell University and currently is working toward her doctorate in Educational Psychology with a specialization in school psychology at the Graduate Center of the City University of New York. Ms. Racanello's research interests include otitis media and its effects on language and learning, attention deficit/hyperactivity disorder's relationship with executive functioning, and managed health care's effect on psychology. She has previously published on otitis media in young children.

Sarah Valley-Gray, PsyD, is an Associate Professor at the Center for Psychological Studies (CPS) at Nova Southeastern University (NSU) in Fort Lauderdale, Florida. Dr. Valley-Gray earned her doctorate in clinical psychology from Nova University. She completed her predoctoral internship with the Division of Psychology, University of Miami/Jackson Memorial Medical Center with an emphasis on pediatric psychology and a school psychology internship in the Dade County Public Schools. She later completed a postdoctoral residency in clinical neuropsychology at NSU. Dr. Valley-Gray is a certified school psychologist in the state of Florida as well as a licensed psychologist. She led the development of the school psychology specialist and doctoral programs at NSU and has demonstrated leadership within the Florida Association of School Psychologists and the National Association of School Psychologists in the areas of training and credentialing. In 2006, she was appointed Director of Continuing Education and Special Projects for CPS. She conducts and publishes research in (1) emergent literacy, (2) pediatric/neurodevelopmental disorders, and (3) training and credentialing issues.

SECTION

I

Schools as Partners in Health Care Delivery

1

Trends in Health Care Delivery

*The Increased Burden on Schools
as Health Care Providers*

Paul C. McCabe and Steven R. Shaw

INTRODUCTION

In addition to teaching basic and advanced academic skills to school-aged children, society asks schools to do significantly more. Schools routinely provide food services, transportation services, liaisons to community services, social services, adult and community education, athletic entertainment, fund raising, research, support for political events, and much more. Most of these activities directly or indirectly affect the teaching and learning of schoolchildren. Despite a lack of formal training, teachers and other educational professionals have branched out into coaching, grant writing, administration, coordination, family counseling, and a host of skills required in the full-service community school (Reeder et al., 1997).

This expansion of teacher roles and skills is born of necessity. However, the largest and most challenging arena that educators are asked to address is medical issues for children.

PEDIATRICS IN THE SCHOOLS

Medical issues in the schools are a reality. At one time, medicine and education were two different professions with very little overlap. Occasionally, a school was required to provide individualized services for children with a chronic illness, or a school building served as a location for community vaccination programs. School-based and school-linked health clinics are located throughout the United States but provide medical services to a small portion of schoolchildren (Brown & Bolen, 2008). U.S. health care has evolved to increase emphasis on access to health care (Shaw, Kelly, Joost, & Parker-Fisher, 1995). Given that 85 million U.S. children between the ages 5 and 19 are mandated to attend school, health care policy and strategies for increasing health access for children and families must involve schools (Clay, Cortina, Harper, Cocco, & Drotar, 2004). Moreover, improvements in health care for school-aged students improve readiness, improve academic achievement, and increase the probability of graduating from high school (Cook, Schaller, & Krischer, 1985). Schools are now integrated components of comprehensive health care delivery for children.

Role of Federal Legislation

Several major federal laws specifically address schools as a location for providing health care. These include the following:

- Americans with Disabilities Act (ADA; 42 U.S.C. § 12101 et seq.) and regulations promulgated by the Department of Justice
- Drug and Alcohol Treatment Records (D&A; 42 USCS § 290dd, 42 CFR 2.1 et seq.)
- Family Educational Right to Privacy Act (FERPA; 20 U.S.C. § 1232g; 34 C.F.R. Part 99)
- Health Insurance Portability and Accountability Act (HIPAA) and regulations adopted under it (45 C.F.R. chapters 160 and 164)
- Individuals with Disabilities Education Improvement Act of 2004 (IDEIA; Public Law 108-446, previously IDEA)
- OSHA Blood-borne Pathogen Standard 29 of C.F.R. 1930.1030
- Prohibition of Mandatory Medication [Child Medication Safety Act (25; Public Law 108-446; Dec. 2004)]
- Proposed New Drug, Antibiotic, and Biological Drug Product Regulations [21 C.F.R. 312.3 (b)]
- Section 504 of the Rehabilitation Act of 1973 (29 U.S.C. § 794)

Moreover, in many states, schools are classified as centers for health care provision for purposes of Medicaid funding. These schools are responsible for compliance with the Medicaid regulations developed by each state. Compliance with legislation, regulation, and case law on educational issues is a complex undertaking. When medical legislation, regulation, and case law are added, the burden on educators can be overwhelming.

Although meeting all the mandates of legislation and case law is a necessity, three major laws affect all schools every day. These are the Individuals with Disabilities Education Improvement Act of 2004, Section 504 of the Rehabilitation Act of 1973, and the Americans with Disabilities Act.

A large portion of school resources is spent attempting to comply with IDEIA, the complex federal funding law for all children receiving special education services. IDEIA requires schools to provide specialized education services and support services (physical therapy, occupation therapy, speech and language therapy, nursing support, and social work support) to children with medical issues that substantially affect learning. All children with special education needs may be eligible to receive these support services. Children receiving special education services under the Other Health Impaired (OHI) category of IDEIA require some form of medical services. The OHI category may include attention deficit/hyperactivity disorder, acute lymphocytic leukemia, meningitis, and a host of other medical conditions. Under IDEIA, schools provide remediation and accommodation for academic issues that are affected directly or indirectly by the long-term effects of a medical issue. Children receiving educational services under the OHI require evidence from a physician of a medical issue that directly impacts academic skill development or academic performance. For children who receive services under OHI, some form of educational collaboration with medical professionals must take place. Moreover, educators must have some degree of understanding as to how the medical issue is likely to affect academic and social issues in order to develop an individualized educational plan.

Section 504 of the Rehabilitation Act of 1973 states that "no otherwise qualified individual with a disability in the United States . . . shall, solely by reason of her or his disability, be excluded from the participation in, denied the benefits of, or be subjected to discrimination under any program or activity receiving Federal financial assistance" (§ 504[a]). Section 504 requires schools to provide accommodations for children with medical issues that may interfere with access to education. Section 504 plans often address educational concerns due to temporary or chronic medical conditions or other medical concerns for which remedial educational services are not required but deviations from the routine scope and sequence of educational curriculum are needed. In addition to other chronic illnesses, drug and alcohol addiction is a health issue covered under Section 504 and must be addressed by schools. Therefore, to provide effective services, teachers and other educational professionals must have some knowledge of the scope, nature, and cause of these medication conditions, as well as the unintended effects of treatment, medications, chronicity, common emotional responses, and related effects on educational functioning.

The Americans with Disabilities Act prohibits discrimination based on disability in employment, state and local government, public accommodations, commercial facilities, transportation, and telecommunications. Schools are required to make reasonable modifications to policies, practices, and procedures where necessary to avoid discrimination, unless they can demonstrate that doing so would fundamentally alter the nature of the service, program, or activity provided. An individual with a disability is defined by the ADA as a person who has a physical or mental impairment that substantially limits one or more major life activities, a person who has a history or record of such impairment, or a person who is perceived by others as having such impairment. Children with chronic illness may be eligible to receive accommodations that require modifications in the physical plant of the school, educational policies, or daily activities in the school setting.

Keeping Pace With the Trends in Health Care

To implement policies and curricula that allow schools to maintain compliance with the myriad laws and regulations, educators must first understand four major domains of knowledge.

The first domain is instruction of students in health literacy, problem solving and communication skills, and promotion of a sense of personal competency and self-efficacy. Health courses, physical education, sex and reproductive health education, and instruction of parents and other family members are common practices in schools. Many aspects of health care instruction include teaching students the behavioral aspects of health care, such as understanding how personal health care decisions are made, avoiding health risk behaviors, and becoming empowered to take control and responsibility for their health care decisions. Many, if not most, schools have developed an effective array of health care education programming for their students and communities.

The second domain is coordination and collaboration with outside agencies, such as public health services, emergency service providers, hospitals, primary care providers, mental health agencies, and dental care providers. Integrating various community agencies to assist schools in meeting their regulatory and legislative requirements concerning health care can be challenging. Health care agencies and schools have different cultures and often have different goals and missions. Health care agencies have their own financial pressures and time limitations. Collaboration between members of the medical and school professions can be difficult. However, it is nearly impossible for educators to meet the increasing health care burden on schools without interdisciplinary collaboration.

The third domain is developing a school environment that promotes healthy living. This includes health care policies, general school rules, supporting effective social environments (e.g., student clubs, volunteerism and associated policies, activities that promote social skills), family support systems, providing healthy role models, effective dietary practice, and the overall development of a healthy school environment. Schools have made major advances in the development of health care policies and promotion of preventative health care practice. Increasingly healthful dietary choices in cafeterias, provision of dietary information to parents, improved antibullying practices, increased quality of physical education programming, promotion of community service, and increased ecological awareness are all approaches taken by schools to advance healthy living.

The fourth domain consists of the physical plant of the school. Lighting, ventilation, noise, sanitation, and other environmental standards all contribute to a healthy environment. In addition, safety standards in the playground, classrooms, and hallways are important to accident prevention. New school construction is increasingly going "green" with substantial improvements in environmental quality and energy efficiency. In fact, almost 1,000 school buildings were considered LEED certified by September 2008; LEED certification means the building met the highest level of energy and environmental performance (USGBC, 2008). Most importantly, knowledge of prevention, treatments, accommodations, and educational implications with regard to medical issues will be of the greatest benefit when implemented in a physical environment that is supportive and healthy for all schoolchildren.

Meeting the Additional Burden

Implementing these laws, plus a variety of statewide regulations concerning health care in the schools, is a complex undertaking. The trend in school-based health care is toward the goals of assessing risks and fostering resilience to ensure that students achieve optimal health, well-being, and academic performance (Kisker & Brown, 1996). To accomplish these ends, multidisciplinary and multiagency collaboration, community support, development of strong policies, dissemination of information, and improving academic achievement are all necessary (Stam, Hoffman, Deurloo, Groothoff, & Grootenhuis, 2006). To be most effective, school-based health care must be

- community based.
- integrated within and supportive of the educational system.
- advised by a school and community group, including parents and students.
- based on accepted standards, regulations, and statutes.
- prepared for crisis management of medical problems.
- supported by a health service management information system.
- capable of providing a range of prevention and treatment services, including those addressing tobacco control, drug and alcohol use, and obesity prevention.
- implemented by sufficient numbers of qualified staff throughout the school day.
- culturally competent and linguistically relevant.
- integrated with educational programming.
- coordinated with the eight components of a comprehensive school health program, as defined by the Centers for Disease Control and Prevention: health education, health services, social and physical environment, physical education, guidance and support services, food service, school and worksite health promotion, and integrated school and community health promotion (Shaw & McCabe, 2008).
- linked with community primary care, regional hospitals, mental health providers, dental providers, local youth- and family-serving agencies, local public health systems, emergency providers, and public insurance outreach programs.
- able to make maximum use of available public and nonpublic funds, such as Medicaid, grants, insurance reimbursement, and business partnerships.
- evaluated regularly to determine effectiveness and efficiency.

Although preventive and primary health care are important parts of school-based health care, medical trends place pressure on schools to provide health care to children with serious illnesses as well. Due to advances in treatment and the necessity of reducing health care costs, children with severe medical issues have fewer inpatient days than in the last decade (Shaw & McCabe, 2008). Whereas many students with conditions such as leukemia, sickle cell anemia, and asthma used to spend many days hospitalized, such children now receive extensive outpatient care and fewer hospitalized days (Kyngas, 2004). This change in the location of medical treatment places more pressures on families and schools. Schools are under increasing pressure to provide homebound instruction, accommodations for medical issues in the classroom, coordination of educational needs with outpatient treatment needs (and the inevitable absences), and preparation for possible emergencies in school settings.

Knowledge of medical issues typically is not part of the curriculum in preparation programs of teachers, psychologists, or other school professionals (Shaw, 2003). Yet legal and regulatory mandates and trends in health care service delivery are placing more responsibility on families and schools. The gap between professional preparation and need for knowledgeable professionals is wide.

2

Collaboration Between Educators and Medical Professionals

Models, Barriers, and Implications

Sarah Glaser, Tia Ouimet, and Steven R. Shaw

Educators have been working with Helena, a 13-year-old student who has been frequently absent from school during the past six months. The school psychologist conducts a diagnostic assessment and determines that the student suffers from generalized anxiety disorder. Helena later reveals that she experiences frequent stomach pains and nausea. Her teachers also report that Helena often asks to be excused from class, either to use the bathroom or visit the school nurse. Her teachers are concerned that, in addition to her anxiety, a medical problem may be causing her pain.

The school psychologist suggests to Helena's family that Helena should see her pediatrician. The pediatrician concludes that there is no physical cause of Helena's stomach pains. When the school psychologist and parents consult with the pediatrician, they both agree that the best course of action is to develop an intervention plan focused on reducing Helena's anxiety. Due to the severity of

Helena's physical symptoms, they agree that she should be monitored by the pediatrician regularly. During a regular follow-up appointment, the pediatrician notes that Helena's stomach pain is still present. He refers Helena and her family to a psychiatrist without first informing the school psychologist. The psychiatrist prescribes antianxiety medication, which requires daily dosage during school hours. Helena's parents do not want their daughter to be labeled as having a mental illness and fear a stigma will be associated with taking medication at school; therefore, they never reveal this information to the school and give Helena the responsibility of taking her medication at school. School-based interventions and medically based interventions are operating independently without communication or coordination.

INTRODUCTION

Nearly 21% of all school-aged children experience behavioral issues that involve medical care, such as attention deficit/hyperactivity disorder (ADHD), depression, and eating disorders, yet nearly two-thirds of these students are not provided with adequate access to treatment (Segool, Mathiason, Majewicz-Hefley, & Carlson, 2009). The same is true for students with chronic medical conditions, such as asthma, juvenile diabetes, and cancer, who make up a total of 15% to 18% of all school-aged children (McCabe & Sharf, 2007). Despite these medical issues affecting school performance there is often lack of collaboration between educators and medical professionals.

Educators and medical professionals are often faced with systemic barriers that may interfere with a collaborative approach to interventions. Understanding the different perspectives and responsibilities of educators and health-care providers is the first step in creating the most appropriate and effective treatment plan (Shaw, Clayton, Dodd, & Rigby, 2004). Within this collaborative framework, long-term strategies to address the inherent differences between the two professions regarding treatment management can be implemented successfully (NASP Delegate Assembly, 2006).

BACKGROUND

Developing a collaborative relationship between school and medical professionals is an important aspect of supporting students with medical and mental health issues and can make a notable difference in their academic performance and overall school experience (Shaw et al., 2004). Although issues of collaboration between educators and medical professionals are not a concern for most students, some do require long-term, ongoing collaboration among educators, the child's family, and medical professionals to receive effective support (Shaw et al.). For example, given that mental health disorders such as ADHD typically involve both medical and educational components, monitoring progress closely and consistently is necessary to ensure adequate collaboration between educators and medical professionals (Shaw & Woo, 2008).

Why Collaboration Between Educators and Medical Professionals Is Necessary

At its best, collaboration among school psychologists, school nurses, teachers, medical professionals, and parents leads to comprehensive treatment for students (Segool et al., 2009). Although school psychologists have a strong training background in the realms of mental health and education, they are not permitted to prescribe medication—a common treatment component for many mental health disorders such as ADHD, autism, anxiety disorders, and depression. However, nearly 55% of all school psychologists are expected to monitor the medication usage of these students, often with little or no communication with the child's psychiatrist. In addition, teachers are responsible for developing the classroom environment and implementing educational interventions. School nurses are often responsible for medication monitoring and administration. Conversely, medical professionals sometimes do not receive adequate information from the school regarding the effects of medication on the function and progress of students (Segool et al.). Coordination of educational professionals within schools is challenging; collaboration with medical professionals outside of the schools is even more complex and difficult.

The overall absence of appropriate collaboration between educators and medical professionals can lead to conflicting treatment plans and decision making without adequate and complete information. Such lapses highlight the need for better service coordination with regards to treatment for children with medical and mental health needs (Segool et al., 2009). Collaborative efforts in treatment planning have the potential to be cost-effective, improve service delivery, avoid duplication of services, and provide a wider variety of service options. Furthermore, consultation between educators and medical professionals can improve working relationships between schools and outside agencies (e.g., hospitals, clinics, and community mental health centers), which in turn can contribute to the student's treatment. Collaboration among professionals can also lead to more positive outcomes for students, such as better academic performance, improved school attendance, increased participation in academic activities, and fewer school disruptions (NASP Delegate Assembly, 2006).

Models of Collaboration

Current models of collaboration for doctors and psychologists in pediatric hospital settings provide a relevant framework for collaboration between educators and medical professionals. Becoming familiar with these working models can be a useful method of learning how to foster cooperation and effective consultation.

Independent Functions Model. The independent functions model is based upon a medical model of consultation, whereby a pediatrician refers a patient to a psychologist for diagnosis and/or treatment (Drotar, 1995). Communication between the pediatrician and psychologist takes place both before and after the referral. Despite this model's efficiency, communication is extremely limited and might not be adequate for students with severe medical or mental health needs. For example, it usually does not provide opportunities to discuss regular progress, alternative treatment options, and clearly defined roles and expectations (Drotar).

Multidisciplinary Team Model. The multidisciplinary model involves several professionals conducting assessments and developing interventions for a single student. In this model, multiple perspectives are developed, yet professionals function in silos. Each professional adds profession-specific skills to the process. For example, teachers address classroom functioning, physicians address medical issues, speech and language pathologists address language issues, and so on. The advantage of this model over the independent functions model is that it considers the complexity of multiple domains of functioning for each student. Yet how these domains interact (e.g., how chronic medical issues might affect attention in the classroom) is not often considered.

Interdisciplinary Team Model. A collaborative interdisciplinary team model, although time consuming and effortful for all individuals involved, may be a better fit for students requiring long-term treatment collaboration between educators and medical professionals. This model involves shared responsibility and decision making among all parties involved in the treatment process, such as school psychologists, doctors, teachers, and school nurses (Drotar, 1995). A collaborative team model encourages consistent and frequent interdisciplinary treatment of the child and allows for educators and doctors to adopt a different perspective on their professional role. For example, school psychologists, teachers, and educators can develop new strategies for identifying the effects of medical issues on students (Drotar). Although this model provides the opportunity for professional growth and teamwork, challenging interprofessional negotiation is required to ensure unique professional contributions are maintained and that organization and leadership are established early in the process (Drotar). The primary difference between the interdisciplinary and multidisciplinary models is that the interdisciplinary model results in one coordinated set of interventions, reached by consensus, and the multidisciplinary model results in multiple interventions, each developed by the specific profession. In this fashion, interactions among medical, psychological, educational, language, and other domains are involved in developing a comprehensive plan.

Transdisciplinary Team Model. The transdisciplinary team model involves the sharing of professional roles and functions. In some descriptions of the transdisciplinary model, professional boundaries are completely blurred. For example, psychologists might conduct a language assessment, a physician might be involved in psychological assessment, and so on. Few professionals are professionally prepared to function in this model. Moreover, legal, professional, and licensing issues make the transdisciplinary model difficult to implement. For example, only physicians are legally allowed to prescribe medications.

Rewards and incentives encourage each professional to operate independently from other professionals. The more collaborative the team model becomes, the more planning, preparation, negotiation, time, and relinquishing of professional autonomy are required. However, this investment pays off in developing increasingly comprehensive interventions.

Obstacles and Barriers to Effective Collaboration

Building and maintaining relationships among medical professionals, educators, and school psychologists is important for all students. However, it is especially important for students with medical and mental health problems. Although the significance of such relationships is recognized, effective collaboration in the school is often difficult because of systemic barriers and interprofessional differences (Shaw et al., 2004; Shaw & Woo, 2008). These barriers can often prevent communication between the school and medical professionals, which leaves the student and the student's family to align medical and school supports on their own (Shaw et al.).

Dual Systems. Physicians and school psychologists, on the one hand, and educators, on the other, use two different—but parallel—systems of diagnosis, service delivery, and treatment (Shaw, Clayton, Dodd, & Rigby, 2009). There are many differences between these systems; however, there are also just enough similarities between the two to create confusion for professionals and parents (Shaw et al.).

One of the main differences between the systems is how they diagnose diseases and disorders. Physicians refer to the *International Classification of Diseases (ICD-10)* and the *Diagnostic and Statistical Manual of Mental Disorders*, text revision (*DSM-IV-TR*; APA, 2000), and psychologists also refer to the *DSM-IV-TR*. Educators, on the other hand, refer to the guidelines outlined in the Individuals with Disabilities Education Act (IDEA), which each state interprets differently according to its individual regulations and which each local educational agency implements separately. An example of the confusion the different diagnostic criteria can create is when a physician diagnoses a learning disability and educators find that the same child is not eligible for the learning disabilities classification within the special education system. Another example is when a physician requests educational assistance for a child with attention deficit/ hyperactivity disorder (ADHD), yet the child's teachers do not believe that these services are appropriate because there is limited evidence that the child's academic performance is impaired by ADHD. Neither the physician nor the educators are wrong in these examples. The physician is making correct diagnoses and treatment recommendations based on *ICD-10* or *DSM-IV-TR*. The educators are correct in using state criteria for disability classification and local procedures to implement IDEA (Shaw et al., 2009).

Interprofessional Tensions. As educators, school psychologists, and physicians continue to specialize and develop new areas of professional expertise, there is an increasing potential for them to step across the professional boundaries of each another (Drotar, 1995). For example, a physician and psychologist may work closely together to provide care for a student with juvenile diabetes. Both professionals can benefit greatly from this collaborative relationship, as the physician can learn practical ways to manage medication adherence issues and the psychologist can learn about individualized management of medication requirements that can be useful in school-based behavioral interventions (Drotar).

Although this blurring of professional roles and boundaries can bring about positive outcomes, it can also create interprofessional conflict and tension. The quality of the collaborative relationship and the level of communication and trust between collaborators is an important component of effective collaboration. If the professionals have a poor relationship and poor communication, then they may feel that their colleagues' behavior is an infringement on their professional roles (Drotar, 1995).

Differences in professional training, tradition, and philosophies can also create conflict between collaborators (Drotar, 1995). For example, the communication styles of a physician can be quite different from those of a psychologist. This can create frustration for parents who are working with both professionals, which in turn can result in a strained relationship between the physician and psychologist.

Finally, interprofessional conflicts can arise as a result of the expectations about professional roles. Collaboration is most effective when professionals of equal status are involved (Power & Blom-Hoffman, 2004). Typically, physicians are of higher social status than educators. Discrepancies between what colleagues expect and how they view their relationship with the other collaborators can be a significant source of tension in the relationship (Drotar, 1995). Because effective collaboration depends on mutual understanding and trust, when mutual expectations are not properly conveyed to all involved in the process, tension can result. Managing expectations concerning status, trust, and equality of decision-making responsibilities is critical to effective collaboration.

Financial and Administrative Issues. There are also financial and administrative barriers to effective collaboration. Physicians are under great pressure to earn revenue to pay for the substantial costs associated with running a medical practice (Shaw & Woo, 2008). Therefore, physicians spend as much of their time as possible engaged in activities that are likely to receive reimbursement from insurance companies and/or government insurance. School visits, collaboration, prevention and promotion programs, and preparatory communication with school personnel are rarely well reimbursed. Schools also feel significant financial pressures, as their budgets are shrinking and, at the same time, their student populations are growing (Shaw &Woo). Dedicating personnel to develop and manage collaborative relationships among educators, school psychologists, and physicians is often not feasible because of these financial and administrative constraints.

Legal Issues. Although there are many laws relevant to health care service delivery in the schools, the Health Insurance Portability and Accountability Act of 1996 (HIPAA) has had the most influence on collaboration between systems. A comprehensive law, HIPAA has several provisions for maintaining privacy of records. Under HIPAA, written parental permission for sharing medical information in a school setting is required. Some parents wish to keep medical issues hidden from school personnel; in such cases, full and complete collaboration between medical and school personnel is not possible.

Credentialing. Each state and province has different sets of credentialing laws and standards regarding the scope of professional practice for educators, physicians, and all other professionals. Responsibility for diagnosis, medication management, and location of service delivery may be restricted in some states.

Ethical Issues. Whenever different professions come together collaboratively, they face special barriers in terms of upholding their professional ethical standards while also maintaining the collaborative relationship (Drotar, 1995). Different ethical standards across different professions can create tension due to this struggle between the need to respect the practices and standards of another profession and the obligation to abide by one's own ethical standards.

IMPLICATIONS FOR EDUCATORS

Strategies for Effective Collaboration
Between Educators and Medical Professionals

Educators and medical professionals can use several strategies to ensure effective collaboration regarding a child's treatment. This cooperative relationship can help professionals develop the most appropriate and comprehensive intervention plan for the student, which in turn can lead to positive treatment outcomes.

Respecting Professional Boundaries. Respecting professional boundaries is a crucial component of effective collaboration between educators and doctors. Although sharing information is an important part of developing treatment plans for students, only the appropriate professional should decide how to apply this knowledge (Shaw et al., 2009). For example, medical professionals should not make school educational placement decisions, and educators should refrain from making medication-based treatment decisions. Educators and medical professionals must also acknowledge the inherent differences in approaches to treatment and delivery of services among all parties involved, while at the same time respecting the expertise of each professional (Benson, Hughes, Helwig, & Shapiro, 2009). Despite the need for professional boundaries, input from all individuals can be beneficial. For example, teachers and school nurses can help guide medical treatment decisions by the child's physician when they notice physical changes in the student, such as stomach pain or nausea with no known origin (Shaw et al.).

Encouraging Active Participation. Although maintaining professional boundaries is a crucial aspect of effective collaboration, encouraging interaction between educators and medical professionals is also important (Shaw et al., 2009). For example, school psychologists and educators can attend a student's appointment with the doctor, and pediatricians can attend a student's school IEP meeting to discuss special services. Taking time out of busy schedules shows commitment to achieving the best possible treatment for the child. In addition, professionals are able to foster cooperative relationships with each other as an interdisciplinary team. Inviting other professionals to review reports or provide insight regarding treatment progress is another way that educators and medical professionals can foster a collaborative relationship (Shaw & Woo, 2008).

Promoting Frequent and Clear Communication. Communication also plays a key role in successful collaboration. Professionals must acknowledge that vocabulary may be domain-specific and that jargon should be avoided to prevent miscommunication. School psychologists, school nurses, hospital-based teachers, and other professionals with experience with both education and medical issues can act as medical-educational liaisons to improve communication between educators and medical personnel (Shaw et al., 2009).

Communication between educators, medical professionals, and parents should be frequent and consistent. All information from release forms, consultation request forms, and collaborative treatment contracts must be completed efficiently (Segool et al., 2009; Shaw et al., 2009). In addition, the nature of the treatment plan and collaboration must be explained to parents in detail before it begins. All agencies involved in the treatment should respond to phone calls and other forms of communication in a timely fashion (Shaw et al.). Making a pamphlet available that outlines school policy regarding collaboration with medical professionals and provides contact information of appropriate staff can be helpful to parents (Shaw & Woo, 2008).

Fostering Community Relationships. Educators can improve collaborative efforts with medical professionals by fostering strong community relationships. For example, they can work with parents and agencies, such as mental health clinics and hospitals, to clarify the needs and available resources both in the community and at the school (NASP Delegate Assembly, 2006). Educators can also develop working relationships with medical personnel by developing a shared goal for collaborative outcomes with regard to service delivery to students. An understanding of each community agency's role can be crucial in addressing service limitations or preventing service duplication. Working with community agencies to create shared protocols that address issues of confidentiality, professional ethics, and referrals sets a tone for further collaboration. Lastly, parents, too, should be encouraged to advocate for active collaboration between educators and medical professionals (Benson et al., 2009).

Developing Prevention and Health Promotion Programs for Students. The development of both prevention programs and health care promotion programs offered through schools benefits students and encourages col-laboration between educators and medical professionals, including school psychologists, school nurses, and pediatricians. Obesity prevention pro-grams, sex education courses, and substance abuse prevention are exam-ples of school-based programs that combine medical and educational knowledge (Shaw & Woo, 2008). The creation and implementation of these programs provides professionals with the opportunity to work together to benefit the outcomes of all students.

Conclusions and Future Directions

Collaboration between educators and health care professionals is essential to supporting students with medical issues. A medical-educational liaison may promote communication between educators and doctors regarding treatment options and can be a valuable addition to many school systems. Although recognizing the importance and valuing the impact of such collaboration, educators and medical professionals often face barriers that prevent the medical-educational liaison role from being effectively established. A necessary first step to collaboration is to understand the systemic barriers to collaboration, as well as the different perspectives and responsibilities of all professionals involved in the collaborative relationship. When these barriers are addressed and overcome, then the fruits of an effective collaborative relationship between the medical and school communities can be realized (Shaw & Woo, 2008). The complex needs of schoolchildren's medical and mental health issues cannot be solved effectively by systems working in isolation.

EDUCATIONAL STRATEGIES

- Respect professional boundaries. Educators must not make medication-based treatment decisions, and doctors must not make decisions regarding school-based interventions or placements.
- Be concise and direct when communicating with medical professionals by developing a few key questions.
- Information shared with medical professionals should be factual rather than based on opinion or judgment.
- Connect with local medical professionals in the community, including pediatricians, clinic staff, and nurse practitioners, to develop working relationships.
- Use a medical-education liaison whenever possible to ensure effective communication. Hospital-based teachers, school nurses, school psychologists, and other professionals who have knowledge of both medicine and education can act as liaisons.
- Invite active participation from medical professionals with regards to treatment plans. For example, the child's pediatrician can attend a school IEP meeting.
- Make a pamphlet available to parents that outlines school policy regarding collaboration with medical professionals and options for parents.
- Develop prevention and health promotion programs (e.g., obesity prevention courses, sex education classes) offered through schools to educate students and encourage collaboration between educators and medical professionals.
- Provide training workshops to parents, teachers, and other school personnel who may not be familiar with how to monitor a child's functioning at home or at school.
- Encourage parents to become advocates for effective communication between educators and medical professionals.

DISCUSSION QUESTIONS

1. What are some of the potential implications of parents withholding important medical information from the school?

2. What steps can schools take to ensure proper communication among educators, parents, and medical professionals?

3. School nurses, educators, school psychologists, physicians, and parents must work closely to monitor students' medication use. What can schools do to foster this collaborative relationship?

4. What are the benefits of providing workshops and information sessions to professionals about proper consultation and collaboration strategies?

RESEARCH SUMMARY

- Nearly 21% of all school-aged children experience behavioral issues that involve medical care, such as ADHD, depression, and eating disorders, yet nearly two thirds of these students are not provided with adequate access to treatment. The same is true for students with chronic medical conditions, such as asthma, juvenile diabetes, and cancer, who make up a total of 15% to 18% of all school-aged children.

- Schools are increasingly acting as the primary mental health provider for the majority of students. However, only a small amount of the available time is spent directly providing these services to students.

- The use of psychotropic medications has increased significantly over the past 10 years. Because of this rise, educators are increasingly required to monitor students' medication use and their behavior.

- The role of a medical-educational liaison—a school psychologist, nurse, or hospital-based teacher who is knowledgeable in both fields—may help promote effective communication between educators and doctors regarding treatment options.

- Many barriers face the collaboration between educators and medical professionals. However, strategies such as clear communication and encouraging community outreach can eliminate some of these obstacles.

RESOURCES

American Academy of Pediatrics—Parenting Corner: www.aap.org/parents.html
Mental Health America (formerly the National Mental Health Association): www.nmha.org
National Association for the Education of Young Children: www.naeyc.org
Atkinson, M., & Hornby, G. (2002). *Mental health handbook for schools.* New York: Routledge Falmer.

Cooley, M. L. (2007). *Teaching kids with mental health and learning disorders in the regular classroom: How to recognize, understand, and help challenged (and challenging) students succeed.* Minneapolis, MN: Free Spirit.

McDermott, D. R. (2008). *Developing caring relationships among parents, children, schools, and communities.* Thousand Oaks, CA: Sage.

Power, T. J., & Blom-Hoffman, J. (2004). The school as a venue for managing and preventing health problems: Opportunities and challenges. In R. Brown (Ed.), *Handbook of pediatric psychology in school settings* (pp. 37–48). Mahwah, NJ: Lawrence Erlbaum.

Weinfeld, R., & Davis, M. (2008). *Special needs advocacy resource book: What you can do now to advocate for your exceptional child's education.* Waco, TX: Prufrock Press.

HANDOUT

STRATEGIES FOR EFFECTIVE COMMUNICATION BETWEEN EDUCATORS AND MEDICAL PROFESSIONALS

- Be aware of the interprofessional differences in assessment, treatment, and service delivery approaches.
- Respect professional boundaries.
- Be concise when communicating by developing a few key questions and summary statements regarding the child.
- Invite participation from other parties. For example, the child's pediatrician can attend a school IEP meeting to discuss intervention plans.
- Information shared with medical professionals should be factual rather than based on opinion or judgment.
- Encourage parents to become advocates for effective communication between educators and medical professionals.

Collaborative Service Delivery Model

Communication among the student's school psychologist, teacher(s), medical professional, and family must be collaborative and ongoing throughout mental health treatment. The goal of this feedback loop is to improve the child's social, emotional, and academic functioning.

School Psychologist
- Communicates with all parties regarding the child's treatment at home and school.
- Creates and monitors school-based intervention plans.

Teacher
- Implements intervention plans in the classroom.
- Consults with school psychologist to monitor impact of classroom-based intervention.

Child's Family
- Involved in planning and management of treatment.
- Consults with school psychologist to monitor impact of home-based interventions.

Medical Professional
- Plans medication-based treatment.
- Communicates with all parties regarding the goals and monitoring of medication-based treatment.

Concepts Adapted From:

Benson, J. L., Hughes, C., Helwig, J., & Shapiro, E. S. (2009). Facilitating relationships with pediatricians. *Communiqué, 37,* 1.

Segool, N. K., Mathiason, J. B., Majewicz-Hefley, A., & Carlson, J. S. (2009). Enhancing student mental health: Collaboration between medical professionals and school psychologists. *Communiqué, 37,* 1–4.

Shaw, S. R., Clayton, M. C., Dodd, J. L., & Rigby, B. T. (2009). Collaborating with physicians: A guide for educators. *Communiqué , 37,* 1–3.

Current Issues in Pediatric Disorders and Treatments

3

Role of Otitis Media in Hearing Loss and Language Deficits*

Amy Racanello and Paul C. McCabe

Jerry is a 5-year-old kindergarten student with a history of chronic otitis media. He often looks flushed. Jerry rubs his cheeks and pulls at his ear lobes on those days when he complains that the side of his head hurts. It is apparent that he is experiencing discomfort, but it is unclear how to help him.

At times, Jerry appears to be inattentive even when the class is engaged in math, which is his favorite subject. When the teacher asks Jerry to repeat the instructions to the class, he is often unable to do so even when he appears to have been paying attention. When the class is watching a movie, Jerry asks for the TV volume to be louder and is observed shifting his chair closer to the TV. When participating in quiet play, Jerry participates appropriately with the other students and plays board games and computer games and creates arts and crafts. However, when on the playground, where it is noisy and there are many distractions, Jerry is not as engaged. He appears to be overwhelmed and unsure of the rules of the games the other children are playing.

Although Jerry's schoolwork is always completed and he is well behaved, the teacher is concerned that he is not getting the full benefit out of his class time.

---

*Adapted from Racanello, A., & McCabe, P. C. (2006). Otitis media: The silent culprit in hearing loss and language deficits. *Communiqué, 35*(2), 32–34. Copyright by the National Association of School Psychologists, Bethesda, MD. Use is by permission of the publisher. www.nasponline.org

He does appear to be attaining the skills he needs to be successful in first grade, including reading and speech skills.

Jerry's parents explain that they frequently take him to the doctor for his ears and they are compliant with the medications. Jerry's mother informs the teacher that he is scheduled to have a myringotomy over the summer between kindergarten and first grade. Although Jerry could have had the myringotomy right away, Jerry's mother is more concerned about him missing school. She also explained that she is concerned about the anesthesia and hopes that he improves before the summer so surgery is not needed.

INTRODUCTION

Ear infection, or otitis media (OM), is the most frequently diagnosed illness among children in the United States (Roberts et al., 2004). Frequent ear infections during the first two years of life can have a deleterious effect on a child's hearing and may lead to impairment of the child's developing language and speech skills. Problems with developing language and speech skills can subsequently lead to academic troubles, including weaknesses in nonword reading, reading fluency, comprehension activities, decoding skills, and mapping phonemes onto graphemes (Winskel, 2006).

BACKGROUND

Disease Overview

Otitis media (OM) is the inflammation of the middle ear, which can be accompanied by the presence of fluid. OM affects 75% to 95% of the pediatric population at least once. Most episodes occur within the first three years of age, with frequency of episodes most likely to peak between 12 to 18 months (Petinou, Schwartz, Gravel, & Raphael, 2001).

In healthy children, the middle space behind the eardrum is filled with air. However, when a child is experiencing an upper respiratory tract infection, the upper respiratory tract, including the middle ear, is congested with mucous. When the middle ear is filled with fluid, the eardrum is not able to vibrate properly, which leads to decreased conduction of sounds and reduced hearing. The hearing deficits persist until the fluid dissipates. Otitis media is often recurrent and varies in degree (Klausen, Moller, Holmefjord, Reisaeter, & Asbojornsen, 2000). When the middle ear is filled with infected fluid, the child's condition is known as acute otitis media (AOM). Symptoms of AOM include fever, irritability, and pain (Zeisel & Roberts, 2003).

Frequently, the fluid in the ear will not become infected, or if the fluid is infected, the infection will spontaneously resolve. Sometimes, however, the fluid will not dissipate. When this occurs, the condition is known as otitis media with effusion (OME), or "glue ear" (Higson & Haggard, 2005). The noninfected fluid may persist for several weeks or even months. If the fluid remains in the child's ear for more than three months, then the condition is considered to be chronic OME.

Medical Treatment

Frequently, children with OME will not be treated unless the fluid becomes infected or if hearing loss is observed. When treatment is required, antibiotic therapy is the most common treatment for acute otitis media. The effectiveness of antibiotic therapy in treating OME is not conclusive; antibiotics have a beneficial but limited effect on treating recurrent otitis media and short-term OME, but longer-term benefits on OME have not been found (Williams, Chalmers, Stange, Chalmers, & Bowlin, 1993). Recent evidence indicates that young children treated with antibiotic medication are more likely to have recurrence of AOM within 3 years (63%) than those children with AOM who did not receive antibiotics (43%; Bezáková, Damoiseaux, Hoes, Schilder, & Rovers, 2009). This means that antibiotic medication should be used judiciously in treating AOM. In fact, when parents are counseled about the course of AOM and cautioned against unnecessary use of antibiotics, more than 63% of parents opt to not treat their children with antibiotics (Pshetizky, Naimer, & Schvartzman, 2003).

In chronic cases of OM, clinicians may recommend that surgery be performed to alleviate the child's chronic ear infections. The surgery, known as myringotomy, requires that a pressure equalization tube (P.E. tube) be placed in the child's middle ear (Zeisel & Roberts, 2003).

Risk Factors for Developing Otitis Media

Multiple factors, including environmental, developmental and biological factors, increase a child's chance for developing OM. Environmental risk factors for developing chronic OM include an episode of otitis media during the first six months of life, parental smoking, infant feeding practices (including bottle feeding and position of the bottle during feeding), socioeconomic status, and group day care attendance (Feldman et al., 2003; Pichichero, 2000; Zeisel & Roberts, 2003). Children who participate in group child care are more likely to develop frequent and recurrent upper respiratory tract infections, which are a major contributor to eustachian tube dysfunction (Zeisel & Roberts). Interestingly, the prevalence of OM is higher in affluent white children, which may be indicative of greater access to medical care and, therefore, greater detection of the disease.

Age. One of the greatest risk factors for developing OME is age (Pichichero, 2000; Zeisel & Roberts, 2003). Children who are younger than age 3 are at an increased risk for OME because their eustachian tubes are more horizontally aligned than those of older children. The horizontal position of the tubes makes it more difficult for fluid to drain from the middle ear. Children commonly experience their first bout of OME by the age of 6 months (Zeisel & Roberts). According to Zeisel & Roberts, "the percentage of children developing at least one episode of OME between the ages of 2 months and 6, 12, and 24 months was 48%, 79% and 91%, respectively" (p. 110).

Chronicity. Chronicity is a risk factor for children who have had their first episode of OM at an early age. These children show a greater risk for developing repeated and/or chronic episodes of OM (Miccio, Gallagher, Grossman, Yont, & Vernon-Feagans, 2001).

Hereditability. There is a hereditable component associated with OM, as children who have had an episode of OM by the age of 6 years are most likely to have maternal history of otitis media (Pichichero, 2000). The likelihood of identical twins or triplets having an ear infection simultaneously is around 60%, whereas the prevalence for fraternal twins is around 30% (Casselbrant et al., 1999). Heritability differs by gender. For example, researchers report that girls show 74% variability in genetic propensity for OM, with the remaining 26% variability due to individual environmental factors. For boys, 45% of the variability is attributed to genetic factors, while 29% is accounted for by common familial environment and 26% by individual environmental factors (Kvaerner, Tambs, Harris, & Magnus, 1997).

Chromosomal Disorders. Several chromosomal disorders cause eustachian tube dysfunction and concomitant OM, including Down syndrome, Williams syndrome, Apert syndrome, fragile X syndrome, Turner syndrome, cleft palate, and autism. Ear examinations of 83% of children with Down syndrome indicate abnormal results, including OM. Of those children with abnormal results, 59% exhibit OME in at least one of their ears (Zeisel & Roberts, 2003). Many children with Down syndrome have stenotic (narrow) external ear canals, which cause eustachian tube dysfunction.

Biofilms. Recent research suggests that bacterial biofilms may be directly contributing to conditions of chronic ear infections (Hall-Stoodley et al., 2006). Biofilms are colonizations of bacteria that attach to surfaces and serve as a defensive barrier for the bacteria. Bacterial biofilms are also antibiotic-resistant. Children with a history of chronic ear infections, including those who are asymptomatic, have been found to have bacterial biofilms on their middle ear tissue. Control subjects who did not have a history of OM do not exhibit biofilms. These results suggest that recurrent OM may be due not to reinfection but rather to persistent biofilms that are metabolically resistant to antibiotics. Although antibiotic therapy is typically effective for those children with acute OM without the presence of biofilms, children with chronic OM typically receive little benefit from antibiotic therapy and are better treated by myringotomy (Hall-Stoodley et al.).

Chronic Allergies. Chronic allergies are a potential risk factor for OM. Allergic rhinitis has been associated with OME, most likely due to the inflammation of the mucosa of the middle ear (Greiner, 2006). Rhinitis can be attributed to airborne allergens, such as pollen, mold, dust, and dander, as well as nonallergic irritants, such as fumes, odors, and smoke. In general, any allergic reaction that leads to mucosa inflammation and fluid accumulation in the middle ear may lead to OME. Food allergies have been suggested as a possible contributory source of chronic OM (Nsouli et al., 1994), but this hypothesis has not been supported by scientific trials using control samples. The pathogenic role of food allergies in OM is likely exceptional, and further research is needed (James, 2004).

Otitis Media: Speech and Language Development

Otitis media with effusion is the most frequent cause of acquired hearing loss in children (Butler, van der Lindern, MacMillian, & van der Wouden,

2003). The link between OME and speech and language development may be related to the fluctuating hearing loss that accompanies OME. The hearing loss may impair the ability to hear certain speech sounds and subsequently process those sounds. The result is that a child with hearing loss may perceive information ineffectively, incompletely, and/or inaccurately (Klausen et al., 2000; Zeisel & Roberts, 2003). Children who experience hearing loss from OM in the early stages of speech development may receive a fluctuating speech signal, which would make it difficult to extract consistent sounds from the speech stream. For example, infants with positive histories of OM have weaker perceptions of phonemes when compared with infants without histories of OM. This could be due to inconsistencies in hearing ability when fluid is present in the middle ear (Polka & Rvachew, 2005). These inconsistencies impede the infant's ability to form well-defined speech and sound categories based on what he or she is hearing. This, in turn, would lead to insensitivity to the phonetic characteristics of sounds and subsequent language and learning weaknesses.

The casual link among OM, hearing, and language development remains equivocal, in part due to methodological limitations of the research. Some studies have found that children who experience OM in early childhood have poorer speech and language skills, specifically articulation and expressive language skills, when compared to their typically developing peers (Klausen et al., 2000; Shriberg, Flipsen, Kwiatkowski, & McSweeny, 2003). In regard to reading, children between 6 and 8 years old with histories of OM and varying degrees of hearing loss demonstrate weaker reading skills and reading delays when compared to children in the same age range without histories of OM (Golz et al., 2005; Kindig & Richards, 2000). Studies have also found higher incidences of teacher-reported behavior problems in children with histories of bilateral OM compared to their age peers. Research indicates that early-onset OM can lead to long-term cognitive deficits, such as sequential information-processing weaknesses found in students over 16 years old (Secord, Erickson, & Bush, 1988). On the other hand, some studies found little or no link between OM and early language development and later academic achievement (Higson & Haggard, 2005; Zeisel & Roberts, 2003).

IMPLICATIONS FOR EDUCATORS

Early OM history and concomitant language deficits are preventable and treatable. Therefore, it is important that educators, especially those working in early childhood classrooms, are knowledgeable about observing behaviors associated with OM in preschoolers. Further, elementary educators need to understand the relationship between a history of chronic OM and later reading and language development (Petinou et al., 2001).

Infants with greater than 20 dB average hearing loss from 12 to 18 months of age have a 33% probability of developing speech disorders at 3 years of age (Shriberg, Friel-Patti, Flipsen, & Brown, 2000). Speech and language secondary symptoms of OM also depend on complex associations with the individual child and environmental variables. When a child presents with a history of OM, his or her speech development should be monitored from as early as 6 months of age (Petinou et al., 2001; Roberts et al., 2004).

Of elementary school students with learning disabilities, 25% experience recurrent ear infections (Reichman & Healey, 1983). Significant differences exist between children with and without early histories of OM. Children aged 6 to 8 years with histories of OM demonstrate significant weaknesses with nonword reading, reading fluency, and comprehension activities and struggle with word decoding skills and mapping phonemes onto graphemes, a skill needed for successful reading (Winskel, 2006).

Student-Specific Strategies

Educators who are knowledgeable of the symptoms that indicate that a child is suffering with OM can help detect the illness early and eventually impact the child's academic performance. Educators in early childhood classrooms are encouraged to pay attention to children showing signs of illness, which will be much more apparent than behaviors that are a result of hearing loss. They should observe if a child

- has a fever;
- pulls on his or her ear;
- complains of ear pain; and/or
- acts in an unusually irritable manner.

When children have been diagnosed with OM, educators can observe if a child is demonstrating behaviors that may result from hearing loss, including if the child does any of the following:

- Struggles with paying attention.
- Demonstrates diminished attention from previous observations.
- Fails to respond when spoken to.
- Sits closer to and/or requests to sit closer to audio stimuli, such as computer and TV speakers.

These behaviors are indirect signs of temporary and/or fluctuating hearing loss associated with otitis media. If a child is demonstrating these signs, educators can recommend a hearing assessment to rule out possible hearing loss. Children who have suffered with OM may exhibit significant weaknesses in reading decoding, fluency, and comprehension skills and should be closely monitored.

General Classroom Strategies

Educators should strive to maintain healthy and clean classrooms. Frequent washing of hands, furniture, supplies, and toys will decrease the spread of contagious respiratory infections and may be helpful in reducing subsequent ear infections.

Educators who promote good listening and healthy hearing practices benefit all children, especially those who experience hearing loss. Educators are encouraged to help children hear and understand speech from others. To facilitate the development of students' listening skills, one should check frequently to make sure children understand what they have heard by asking them to retell what they heard in their own words.

Additionally, one can decrease background noise by limiting exposure to and/or eliminating noisy toys from the classroom, closing windows and doors, creating quiet areas/centers in the classroom, and using dividers in play areas and centers. These measures will minimize distractions for children when they need to listen.

Language learning strategies, such as reading stories aloud to children, creating a literacy-rich classroom, giving books and magazines to children to look at on their own, and supplying visual aids such as maps and pictures, will help facilitate literacy learning for all children.

EDUCATIONAL STRATEGIES

- Is a child demonstrating behaviors that may result from hearing loss? Indirect signs of temporary and/or fluctuating hearing loss associated with otitis media include difficulty paying attention, diminished attention, not responding when spoken to, and requesting to and/or sitting closer to audio stimuli, such as speakers.
- Is a child showing signs of illness? Such signs will be more noticeable than behaviors that are a result of hearing loss. Observe if the child has a fever, pulls on an ear and/or complains of ear pain, or acts unusually irritable.
- If children have developmental and/or environmental risk factors associated with OM, have a history of OM, or demonstrate behaviors associated with hearing loss, educators or parents can recommend a hearing assessment.
- Decrease background noise to minimize distractions for children when they need to listen, limit students' exposure to noisy toys, create quiet areas/centers in the classroom, and arrange dividers for small-group play and reading.
- To help children hear and understand speech, ensure they are within three feet of the listener and standing still when speaking. Frequently check to make sure students understand what has been said by asking them to retell the content in their own words.
- Read stories aloud to children; give students books and magazines to look at on their own; read about and discuss daily experiences, such as media headlines; and supply students with visual aids, such as charts, maps, and pictures.

DISCUSSION QUESTIONS

1. What intervention strategies can be used to help educators and parents of children with OM? Give specific examples of each.

2. Both environmental and biological factors can increase a child's risk for developing OM. What role can educators take in encouraging parents to examine these factors and perhaps make changes to lessen the number of infections? What can be done in the school environment to reduce the number of infections?

3. Children who have positive OM histories are at possible risk for learning difficulties. Why do you think this is, and how can this be prevented once the child is in school?

4. When a child has a history of OM, what other professionals should be consulted when planning the child's education? Why? What role do educators have in coordinating among these professionals?

RESEARCH SUMMARY

- Despite research limitations, sufficient data have been aggregated supporting the link between early OM history and language deficits later in life.
- OM cases have been documented to be twice as common in students with learning disabilities as in students without learning disabilities. Of elementary school students with learning disabilities, 25% experience recurrent ear infections.
- Significant differences exist in the reading development of children with and without early histories of OM. Children with histories of OM demonstrate significant weaknesses with nonword reading, reading fluency, comprehension, word decoding skills, and mapping phonemes onto graphemes—all skills that are needed for successful reading.
- When a child presents with a history of OM, his or her speech development should be monitored from as early as 6 months of age.
- Infants with greater than 20 dB average hearing loss from 12 to 18 months of age have a 33% probability of developing subclinical (i.e., emergent) and clinical speech disorders by 3 years of age. The speech and language secondary symptoms of OM also depend on complex associations with the individual child and environmental variables, such as duration and chronicity of OM, access to medical care, and response to treatment.

RESOURCES

American Speech-Language-Hearing Association (ASHA). (2008). *Hearing assessment.* Retrieved September 19, 2009, from http://www.asha.org/public/hearing/testing/assess.htm

Block, M. A. (1998). *No more amoxicillin: Preventing and treating ear and respiratory infections without antibiotics.* New York: Kensington.

Centers for Disease Control and Prevention (CDC). (2009). *Get smart: Know when antibiotics work.* Retrieved September 19, 2009, from http://www.cdc.gov/getsmart/

National Institute on Deafness and Other Communication Disorders (NIDCD). (2008). *Ear infections: Facts for parents about otitis media.* Retrieved September 19, 2009, from http://www.nidcd.nih.gov/health/hearing/otitismedia.asp

Schmidt, M. A. (2004). *Childhood ear infections: A parent's guide to alternative treatments.* Berkeley, CA: North Atlantic.

HANDOUT

OTITIS MEDIA

Ear infection, or otitis media (OM), is the most frequently diagnosed illness among children in the United States. Recurrent ear infections during the first 2 years of life can have a harmful effect on a child's hearing and may lead to impairment of the child's developing language and speech skills, which in turn can lead to academic problems.

- What is otitis media?
  - Otitis media is the inflammation of the middle ear.
  - Acute otitis media occurs when the middle ear is filled with infected fluid. This condition is commonly known as an ear infection.
- What risk factors increase a child's chance for developing otitis media?
  - Environmental risk factors for developing chronic OM include an episode of otitis media during the first 6 months of life, parental smoking, infant feeding practices (including bottle feeding and position of the bottle during feeding), and group day care attendance.
  - Age is one of the greatest risk factors for developing chronic ear infections. Children who are younger than age 3 are at increased risk for OME because their eustachian tubes are more horizontally aligned than those of older children.
  - Chronicity is another risk factor. Children who have had their first episode of OM at an early age show greater risk for developing repeated and/or chronic episodes.
  - Chromosomal disorders can cause eustachian tube dysfunction and concomitant OM. These disorders include Down syndrome, Williams syndrome, Apert syndrome, fragile X syndrome, Turner syndrome, cleft palate, and autism.
- What are the effects of otitis media?
  - An ear infection can cause severe pain.
  - An untreated infection can travel from the middle ear to nearby parts of the head, including the brain.
  - Untreated otitis media may lead to permanent hearing impairment.
  - Persistent fluid in the middle ear and chronic otitis media can reduce a child's hearing at a time that is critical for speech and language development.
  - Children who have early hearing impairment from frequent ear infections are more likely to have speech and language disabilities, which can cause later academic problems.
- How can someone tell if a child has otitis media?
  - Otitis media can be a challenge to discover, because most children affected by this disorder are under 3 years old and do not have sufficient speech and language skills to explain what is bothering them. A child with otitis media might demonstrate these common signs:
    - The child may be uncharacteristically irritable.
    - The child may have difficulty sleeping.
    - The child may tug or pull at one or both ears.
    - The child may have a fever.
    - Fluid may drain from the ear.
    - The child may have a loss of balance.
    - The child may be unresponsiveness to quiet sounds and/or show other signs of hearing difficulty, such as being unresponsive, being inattentive, and/or sitting too close to the television.
- Can anything be done to prevent otitis media?
  - While direct prevention strategies are currently not available, environmental risk factors, which make children more susceptible to the illness, can be lessened or eliminated.
    - Environmental tobacco smoke should be avoided.

○ Certain infant feeding practices, including bottle feeding, feeding lying down, and leaving the bottle in the crib with the child during feeding, make children more at risk for otitis media.
○ Children who participate in group child care are more likely to develop frequent and recurrent upper respiratory tract infections, which are a major contributor to ear infections. Children who attend day care should avoid contact with ill playmates.

- How is otitis media treated?
  ○ Antibiotic therapy is the most common treatment for acute otitis media. However, the effectiveness of antibiotics in treating ear infections is not certain, and recurrent use of antibiotic therapy may actually make the child more susceptible to future ear infections.
  ○ In persistent cases, doctors may recommend surgery to alleviate a child's chronic ear infections. The surgery, known as myringotomy, places a pressure equalization tube in the child's middle ear.

- How does otitis media effect speech and language development?
  ○ When children have episodes of otitis media in the early stages of development, they do not hear consistent speech sounds, making it difficult for them to imitate and reproduce accurate speech sounds.

- Some tips to help identify a possible ear infection include the following:
  ○ Observe the child for behaviors that may be the result of hearing loss. Behaviors include having difficulty paying attention or showing diminished attention, not responding when spoken to, and sitting closer to computer and TV speakers.
  ○ Observe the child for symptoms of an ear infection. When a child has an ear infection, the signs of illness will include running a fever, pulling at one or both ears, being irritable, and complaining of ear pain.

- Intervention ideas
  ○ Young children with a history of ear infections or risk for ear infections should have their speech and hearing monitored. A complete audiological assessment provides detailed information about any hearing loss and can be completed in addition to a hearing screening; these are usually coordinated through the pediatrician's office.
  ○ Always promote a healthy environment. Wash hands and toys frequently. Remember that secondhand cigarette smoke increases a child's chance of getting middle ear infections.
  ○ Promote good listening. Help children hear and understand speech and decrease background noise. Encourage children to stand within three feet of the listener before speaking and to stand still to decrease distractions. An example of how to decrease background noise is limiting children's exposure to noisy toys and media.
  ○ Ensure good listening. Frequently check to make sure children understand what they have been told by asking them to retell the content in their own words.
  ○ Promote language learning activities. Ask children simple questions, listen to what they have to say, and talk about topics of interest. You can add to what a child is saying by using more words, praise the child for talking even when speech is unclear, and encourage children to use their words to talk to one another.
  ○ Promote literacy learning. Help children interact with books, songs, and games. Read stories aloud to children. When you read, describe and explain accompanying pictures and refer to the child's own experiences. Give children books and magazines to look at on their own. Read aloud common daily experiences, such as traffic signs, newspaper headlines, and labels on packages.

4

Childhood Immunizations*

The Power of Misinformation

Michelle Klein Brenner and Paul C. McCabe

The following is a true occurrence. The names have been changed to protect the family's identity.

David and Jane are married and have three children. Their children are selectively immunized. This means that David and Jane considered the risks of contracting a disease and their children's ability to withstand it before deciding whether to immunize. Their home state of California allows for personal exemptions of vaccinations, so the children could still attend school.

In January, the family traveled to Europe. When they returned home, their 7-year-old son, John, was not feeling well and stayed home from school for a few days. The day after his return to school, John developed a rash. His mother took him to two different doctors, where he sat in the waiting rooms of each until it was his turn to be seen. As his rash spread and his fever rose, he was sent to two different departments of the hospital for further testing. John was diagnosed with the measles, a disease his parents had chosen not to protect him against. Their choice affected 11 other children.

John's two siblings contracted the disease. On the few days John had attended school, he had infected two other nonimmunized children. His visits to the doctors' offices resulted in the infection of four other children who were in the waiting room with him. One of the children whom John had directly exposed to the illness then infected one of his siblings. John's own siblings infected two additional children. The friends John infected at school passed the disease to three other playmates. Thus, in less than a month, John's contraction of a serious

*Adapted from Klein, M., & McCabe, P. C. (2005). Childhood immunizations: Myths and misconceptions. *Communiqué, 34*(4), 34–35. Copyright by the National Association of School Psychologists, Bethesda, MD. Use is by permission of the publisher. www.nasponline.org

disease affected 11 other children. Some of those children were infected because their parents had made the same choice as David and Jane; others, such as three of the four infected in the waiting room at the pediatrician's office, were infants under the age of 12 months who were not scheduled to receive the MMR immunization for another few months. Over 70 people were quarantined; one infant had traveled on an airplane before developing symptoms, and all the passengers on that flight needed to be notified as well.

INTRODUCTION

Negative effects associated with immunizations and vaccinations have recently garnered much media attention. An understanding of the history of vaccines, the diseases they aim to protect, and the misconceptions associated with them is necessary for parents to make informed decisions for their children, as well as for educators to provide appropriate guidance and assistance in helping parents make these decisions.

BACKGROUND

Development of Vaccinations

In 1776, Dr. Edward Jenner successfully demonstrated that injecting extract from cowpox ulcers resulted in immunity against the smallpox virus (Lochhead, 1991). A century ago, the U.S. infant mortality rate and the childhood mortality before the age of 5 were each 20% (Stern & Markel, 2005), just under 3 times the current rate (Mathews & MacDorman, 2007). Twenty-four years after Jenner's breakthrough, vaccinations were implemented in the United States, and 100,000 individuals in Europe had received the smallpox vaccination (Stern & Markel). The smallpox vaccine was required by law in the United States and Europe during the 19th century. As vaccinations for diphtheria, tetanus, and pertussis (DTP) and measles, mumps, and rubella (MMR) were developed, these immunizations were required for public school attendance. At one time, parents dreaded the thought of their child contracting a disease such as measles or rubella because they had witnessed the devastating effects of the disease firsthand. Today's generation of parents has not had the same experience and, consequently, may question the effects and risks of immunization, stirred on by Internet myths, rumors, media generalizations drawn from extremely rare cases of vaccination reactions, and pseudoscientific claims regarding the causal effects of immunizations (Stern & Markel). As a result, despite years of medical advances that have made protection against debilitating childhood diseases accessible, parents may refuse to immunize their children.

Opposition to Immunization

Fear of Side Effects. Although some religious opposition to immunization exists (Novotny et al., 1988; Peel, 2004), most opposition is due to philosophical reasons. Unfortunately, many of these personal philosophies are based on false assumptions. For example, some individuals believe that receiving vaccinations ultimately weakens the immune system (Gellin, Malbach, & Marcuse, 2000). Others are of the opinion that debilitating side effects emerge. Medical science has refuted both beliefs. The likelihood of contracting an infection does not increase, because modern vaccines have fewer antigens than earlier versions. In fact, failure to immunize a child leaves him or her more vulnerable to an infection than if vaccinated (Offit et al., 2002). In addition, research has indicated that side effects are so rare that they cannot be attributed to the vaccine (e.g., 1 in 450,000 reported an immediate allergic reaction; 1 in 8,000,000 reported a potentially life-threatening reaction; Zent, Arras-Reiter, Broeker, & Hennig, 2002). Modern vaccine production and administration no longer utilize the transfer of fluids from human to human (Bazin, 2003), so the only possible side effects include local redness, irritation, and, in some cases, a mild fever lasting only a few days (Gruber, Nilsson, & Bjorksten, 2001). The majority of doctors assert that the benefit of protecting children from contacting one of these diseases outweighs the mild side effects that may or may not occur due to vaccination (Zent et al., 2002).

Fear of Developing Another Disorder. The most recently publicized reason some individuals choose not to vaccinate their children is the assertion that immunizations result in the development of other disorders. The assertions are specific as to which vaccine is conjectured to cause which disorder.

Hemophilus influenza B (Hib) Vaccine and Diabetes. Hemophilus influenza B is a strain of the flu that affects humans almost exclusively. It begins similarly to a cold; bacteria enter through the nose and mouth and colonize. If it remains in that area of the body, then the symptoms are similar to those of a severe cold. However, the bacteria often spread to the lungs and bloodstream, causing meningitis, pneumonia, and ear infections. Through decades of antibiotic use, bacteria strains have mutated and become more resistant to antibiotics. Vaccination against Hib is extremely important, as children under the age of 5 are most susceptible to contracting the disease and the results can be fatal. Before the vaccine became widespread, Hib meningitis was the most common cause of non-birth-related intellectual disabilities in children. The recommended schedule of the vaccine is at 2 months, 4 months, and 6 months with a booster shot between 12 and 15 months (AAP, 2008).

Some parents neglect to immunize their children against Hib because they believe it causes diabetes. The reasoning behind this claim emerged when the administration of the vaccine in a few children instigated an attack on insulin-producing beta cells in the pancreas similar to Type 1 diabetes (Dinsmoor, 1998). When the remaining cells cannot produce enough sugar-regulating insulin, diabetes emerges. However, confirmatory research does not support this claim. Doctors and researchers believe that the theory probably emerged when children who were already in the prediabetic state were immunized and then developed diabetes (Dinsmoor). Failure to immunize the child would not be the correct solution. In fact, it would be beneficial to introduce this particular immunization at an earlier age before all pancreatic cells were completely developed. This would serve to stop the inflammatory process before it began. It is important to reiterate that this inflammatory process occurs only in those children who are already prediabetic. No causal relationship between any vaccine and diabetes has been established.

Pertussis Vaccine and Asthma. Pertussis, also known as whooping cough, is spread through bacteria leaving the mouth or nose of an infected person and entering that of a healthy person. It begins 3 weeks after exposure, with the symptoms of a cold lasting for about 2 weeks before becoming more serious. A severe cough emerges; during coughing spells, the individual makes a "whoop" sound as he or she struggles to breathe. The individual may also have blue lips and nails as a result of limited oxygen. Complications include seizures, ear infections, and swelling of the brain; the disease can be fatal. Young children are the most susceptible to the disease and often contract it from their parents or older siblings. Immunization is recommended for individuals of all ages, especially those who come into contact with infants. Recently, the pertussis vaccine has received the celebrity endorsement of the actress Keri Russell. Ms. Russell is making every attempt to educate adults, especially parents of infants, about the importance of getting immunized or receiving a booster shot in an effort to protect their children from contracting the disease from their own parents. According to the recommended vaccine schedule, the pertussis vaccine is given in combination with the vaccines for diphtheria and tetanus and is, thus, commonly known as DTaP. Based on the recommended schedule, DTaP is given in five doses, at 2 months, 4 months and 6 months, followed by booster shots between 15 and 18 months and again between 4 to 6 years of age (AAP, 2008). The vaccine does not provide lifelong immunity; therefore, older children and adults should get booster shots every 10 years. Parents of school-aged children should also be especially careful, as the disease often spreads in day care and schools.

Some parents refuse to immunize their children against pertussis based on erroneous information that it causes asthma. There is absolutely no research to support this claim. Numerous studies have been conducted, and no causal link has been identified (Maitra, Sherriff, Griffiths, & Henderson, 2004; Sundqwist, Trollfors, & Taranger, 1998). In fact, given the breathing difficulties brought about by a bout of pertussis, it would seem more likely that asthmalike symptoms might persist following the illness; the DTaP vaccination could prevent these breathing difficulties from ever developing.

Measles, Mumps, Rubella (MMR) Vaccine and Autism. These three diseases are often linked because the vaccine is most readily available in a combination form. The diseases are spread when an individual is exposed to an infected person, especially if that infected person coughs or sneezes. They differ in terms of their specific symptoms.

Measles is highly contagious; when an infected person coughs or sneezes, the bacteria remain in the air for up to 2 hours. A fever develops 1 to 2 weeks after exposure. After approximately another week, a cough develops, and the individual suffers from red, watery eyes and white spots inside the cheeks. A rash spreads throughout the body. Individuals of any age can contract the disease, but children under the age of 5 are most susceptible. Complications include blindness, ear infection, pneumonia, and infection of the brain. When they occur, fatalities are usually due the complications, not the disease itself.

Mumps can be spread by individuals who are unaware that they are infected with the disease; symptoms appear 2 to 3 weeks after infection. The primary symptoms are extremely swollen salivary glands. Other symptoms include fever and pain while chewing or swallowing. Complications include meningitis and hearing loss. Men and teenage boys who contract the disease can suffer from orchitis, a swelling of the testicles that can cause sterility.

Rubella is the mildest of the three diseases. Symptoms begin with a mild fever for a few days, swollen lymph nodes behind the ears, and a rash that spreads from the face downwards. It is highly important that pregnant women are immunized against rubella, as the virus can easily pass to the fetus, resulting in intellectual disabilities, heart malformation, and eye malformation.

Children between the ages of 5 and 9 are most often affected by mumps and rubella, making the vaccine imperative for school-aged children. According to the immunization schedule, the MMR vaccine is recommended between 12 and 18 months of age, with a booster between 4 and 6 years of age (AAP, 2008).

The controversy surrounding the MMR vaccine is due to a claim that it causes autism. In 1998, a study published in *Lancet*, a British journal, followed 12 patients with bowel problems. The study stated that the problems might have resulted from an MMR vaccine (Wakefield et al., 1998). Bowel problems led to decreased absorption of vitamins and nutrients, and this dietary malnourishment was hypothesized to lead to autism. The publication of this study was considered explosive at the time; never before had research indicated any sort of causal link. Six years later, however, 10 of the 13 original researchers had withdrawn their claims (Brown, 2008). The *Lancet* published a retraction of the original study. Despite this and the fact that no relationship has been subsequently found among autism, inflammatory bowel disease, and the MMR vaccination (Fombonne, 1999), the original publication was sufficient to cause parents alarm, and some have elected not to vaccinate their children. In 2000, the American Academy of Pediatrics assembled a panel of multidisciplinary experts to review current research and hypotheses. The consensus was that despite the claims of those who have reached conclusions based on personal experience, no evidence exists of an association between the MMR vaccine and autism or other pervasive developmental disorders or irritable bowel disease (Halsey & Hyman, 2001). Recent investigations indicate that Wakefield falsified data in the original study of the 12 patients (Deer, 2009).

Despite the contradictory evidence, the belief that the MMR vaccine may cause autism continues, in large part due to the efforts of scientists such as Bernard Rimland. Dr. Rimland, a psychologist whose son has been diagnosed with autism, made revolutionary gains in the study of autism. When his child was born in 1956, autism was not a well-known disorder. The prevailing attitude at the time, based on the work of psychologist Bruno Bettelheim, was that the cause of autism was "refrigerator mothers" (i.e., mothers who were so cold and detached that their children needed to withdraw into themselves for comfort). Rimland, however, refuted this notion and did extensive research of his own; he eventually concluded that autism was a neurological disorder, which he believed was caused by mercury. Vaccines at the time contained thimerosal, a mercury-based preservative. Although this theory was met with skepticism (Nelson & Bauman, 2003) and thimerosal was not found to cause harm except for local hypersensitivity reactions (Ball, Ball, & Pratt, 2001), the Food and Drug Administration had thimerosal removed from all routine childhood vaccines in 1999 on the basis that its use provided infants with more mercury than was recommended (Kimmel, 2003).

Personal anecdotes, however, tend to resonate more with parents and other individuals than research statistics. When celebrities like Jenny McCarthy and Holly Robinson Peete use the media to advocate against vaccinating children, parents may make immunization decisions without being fully informed. There should be no attempt to minimize the angst that parents, celebrity or otherwise, experience when told that their child has a diagnosis of autism. Other facts, however, need to be discussed as well. Autism generally becomes most identifiable after a child's first birthday; this coincides with the same time that the MMR vaccine is scheduled. The simultaneous occurrence of these two events may lead parents to associate them. Retrospective research utilizing home videotapes shows that while autism is often diagnosed well after the first birthday, signs and symptoms of social and communication problems, such as failure to make eye contact and not responding to name, are evident before 12 months and, therefore, *before* the administration of the MMR vaccine (Osterling & Dawson, 1994). The existence of symptoms before the child was vaccinated eliminates the causal relationship.

Congress created the National Vaccine Injury Compensation Program in 1988 to investigate allegations of side effects from the diphtheria, tetanus, and pertussis vaccine that was used at the time (HRSA, 2008). Recently, Omnibus Autism Proceedings were held; these special hearings investigated the allegation that children developed autism because of vaccines. One case that came before the court was that of Hannah Poling, a child with a mitochondrial disorder. Hannah, aged 9, had received her vaccinations when thimerosal was still being used. When she was 19 months old, Hannah received five shots to immunize her against nine diseases on the same day in an effort to make up for missed doctor appointments. The court concluded that the stress of receiving the immunizations had aggravated her current condition, resulting in autism-like symptoms, and awarded monetary compensation. When this case was reported upon in the media, it was presented as evidence for those who believe vaccines cause autism; in fact, the opposite is true. The court did not conclude that her symptoms occurred because of the vaccine; rather, the court concluded that her pre-existing mitochondrial disorder in combination with the vaccine resulted in autism-like symptoms (Offit, 2008). For a child like Hannah, any additional stress, such as dehydration or fever, can have negative consequences. The extent to which this case was hyperbolized in the media illustrates how misinformation can propagate.

One final theory related to the autism-vaccine debate exists: that it is the combination of the three vaccinations that is problematic, not each vaccine individually. Concerned parents could request that their pediatricians administer the vaccine in three separate doses. It is important to understand that extensive research has been conducted in this area and no causal link has ever been established between the combined MMR vaccine and autism. The Centers for Disease Control and Prevention (CDC) is conducting ongoing research in this area but to date has not identified a link between the vaccine and autism.

IMPLICATIONS FOR EDUCATORS

The CDC and the state Departments of Health have immunization requirements for student admission to school. To stay in compliance, school administrators and educators should have a plan in place to assist those parents who are hesitant to immunize their children. Educators are in the unique position of being able to fulfill their role as child advocates by explaining the misconceptions associated with vaccinations. In addition, physicians may be too busy to allocate the time needed to explain the benefits of immunizations and any adverse effects to worried parents.

Schools have several options to provide parents with information about immunizations. Schools can provide parents who come to school to register their child or to inquire about registration with a handout or pamphlet addressing the myths related to vaccinations and the importance of immunizing their child. Schools can also organize meetings for community parents to explain the reasons for receiving vaccinations. Perhaps the most important and useful tool educators can provide a parent is time. Educators who are knowledgeable in this area can make themselves available to respond to parents' questions and concerns related to vaccines.

EDUCATIONAL STRATEGIES

- Educators and other support staff advocate for students and students' health. Educators help to ensure that a child is not putting him- or herself and others at risk by failing to receive immunizations. If a nonimmunized child contracts a disease, then he or she can then spread it to other nonimmunized children.
- Educators and school administrators need to be aware of the state policy regarding philosophical, religious, and medical exemptions.
- Educators, administrators, and support staff should educate themselves regarding the myths associated with particular vaccines; this knowledge will allow them to have an informed response when approached by a parent. Professional development workshops can be organized to ensure that school staff is aware of current research. Very often, parents are exposed to misinformation through the Internet and mass media. Their fears and concerns may be stemming from erroneous information. Schools can help ensure that the parent can differentiate between credible and noncredible sources of information in the future.
- Educators and school staff should encourage parents to meet with their pediatricians to discuss concerns. Their physicians have knowledge of medical and scientific information that can help alleviate parents' fears.
- Respect the parent. Independent of what one's personal beliefs may be, a parent who states that he or she does not want to immunize a child due to personal beliefs is likely afraid of the effects. Although

no research supports claims that vaccines cause other conditions, the parent's fear is real and should not be dismissed. Educators and school staff should take the time to discuss the information with the parent.

DISCUSSION QUESTIONS

1. Misinformation about vaccines persists in spite of contrary scientific evidence. What can educators and school support staff do to counteract negative anecdotal stories and allay the parents' fears regarding inoculating their children?

2. Independent of CDC and state health department requirements, do educators and school support staff have any right to sway a parent's decision regarding immunizations?

3. How can educators and school support staff address concerns of parents who do choose to immunize their child regarding those children who receive exemptions to immunizations?

4. Does a school have the right to refuse to provide an immunization exemption to a child? Should medical, religious, and personal exemptions be considered differently?

RESEARCH SUMMARY

- The only scientifically validated side effects of vaccinations are local redness, irritation, and a mild fever.
- A century ago, before the introduction of vaccines, the mortality rate of children under 5 was approximately 3 times the rate it is today.
- The following illnesses are wrongly associated:
  - Hib and diabetes: Research shows that Hib may trigger a diabetic reaction but only in children who are already in a prediabetic state.
  - Pertussis and asthma: No link has ever been established.
  - MMR and autism: This is an area with a vast amount of research. No link exists.

- There are numerous reasons that the unsupported link between MMR and autism exists:
  - A British medical journal published a scientific article reporting a link. These findings were highly publicized. However, the results were never replicated, most of the original authors retracted the findings, and there is evidence that the original results were fabricated.
  - The MMR vaccine is administered at the same time that autism symptoms emerge, implying a connection. However, the correlation is simply due to timing, not causation.
  - Personal anecdotes from celebrities and other parents provide heartbreaking and sensational stories, which the media often presents without medical sources or review.

RESOURCES

Offit, P. A. (2008). *Autism's false prophets: Bad science, risky medicine, and the search for a cure.* New York: Columbia University Press. Dr. Paul Offit wrote this book addressing the inaccuracies of the link between autism and the MMR vaccination.

Sears, R. (2007). *The vaccine book: Making the right decision for your child.* New York: Little Brown. Dr. Robert Sears wrote this book providing information about each vaccine in the childhood immunization schedule, as well as a suggested alternate immunization schedule.

The following valid Web sites provide information on vaccines and the diseases they prevent:

Parents of Kids with Infectious Diseases (PKIDS): www.pkids.org

VaccinePlace: www.vaccineplace.com

HANDOUT

CHILDHOOD IMMUNIZATIONS: KNOW THE FACTS

In today's age of television and the Internet, we are exposed to a steady stream of information and misinformation. Parents of infants and school-aged children bear an enormous responsibility regarding their decision to immunize their children. This has immediate consequences for public health and safety, as diseases proliferate in conditions where vaccinations are unavailable or declined. For this reason, it is most important for parents to educate themselves about this topic from reliable scientific sources.

- Make an appointment with your child's pediatrician for the sole purpose of speaking with him or her regarding your concerns about vaccinations. This will allow you the opportunity to talk without feeling rushed. Make a list of questions or topics and bring it with you to the appointment.
- Look at alternatives before entirely eliminating a vaccine. For example, separating the measles, mumps, and rubella (MMR) vaccine into three discrete doses reduces effectiveness slightly but eliminates the concern of exposing your child to too much vaccine at once. It is certainly a better route than opting out entirely.
- Do not take all information you read or hear at face value. Information without research support is too readily available and can result in misinformed decisions regarding your child. For example, you may find information about the negative effects of mercury contained in vaccines; however, vaccines have not contained mercury since 1999.
- The fact that immunizations do not guarantee long-term immunity is not a reason not to vaccinate a child. Placing a seatbelt on a child does not guarantee that the car will not be in an accident, yet most parents would never fail to secure their child. This holds true in relation to protection against preventable diseases as well.
- Educate yourself using only credible, verifiable sources of information.

5

Shaken Baby Syndrome*

Immediate and Long-Term Consequences and Implications for Educators

Tiffany Folmer Lawrence and Paul C. McCabe

Payton is an 11-year-old who attends a public school. Payton is blind in both eyes and deaf in one ear, and his intellectual ability is severely delayed. He is classified as a student with Multiple Disabilities. He has received special education services since he was 2 years old. Payton's mother, Jacqueline (age 27), indicated that Payton was hospitalized at 3 months old with lethargy, fever, and feeding issues. The doctors diagnosed him as being in septic shock, with probable seizurelike activity. Jacqueline reported that the doctors were not able to predict his prognosis. She reported that Payton's blindness and deafness began after this hospitalization. Payton's developmental milestones were delayed. She reported that Payton has not had contact with his father since he was 6 months old, as he was physically abusive to Jacqueline and she cut off contact from him.

Payton's teacher describes him as a sweet boy who loves to listen to stories, play with animals, and collect things. She shares that he can identify all the letters and numbers using a Braille system. He is able to identify coins by touch, but she struggles with the best method to teach him other life skills, like cooking and mobility, due to safety concerns. She reports that he exhibits inattention, hyperactivity, aggression toward other students and staff, and difficulty handling stress. She wonders if more could be done to help him with regulating his emotions and behavior and to help him improve his safety in the community. She states that he has spent a "lot of time" in the principal's office and that his

*Adapted from Folmer, T., & McCabe, P. C. (2003). Shaken Baby Syndrome: Implications for school psychologists. *Communiqué, 32*(1), 38–41. Copyright by the National Association of School Psychologists, Bethesda, MD. Use is by permission of the publisher. www.nasponline.org

"mother is supportive but stressed beyond belief" trying to cope with his behavioral difficulties, along with being a single mother and working two jobs to pay for Payton's extensive and expensive medical care and outside therapies.

INTRODUCTION

The roles of school mental health professionals are expanding beyond secondary and tertiary intervention to include primary prevention efforts aimed at thwarting trauma and abuse of children. Educators, in addition to medical health and mental health professionals, are required by legal and ethical mandates to report suspected cases of maltreatment. To do so, the mandated reporters need to be knowledgeable of the signs and symptoms of possible abuse, as well as associated risk factors. One form of child abuse, shaken baby syndrome (SBS), has been receiving an increasing amount of attention, both in terms of research focus and media awareness.

BACKGROUND

Shaken baby syndrome occurs when someone shakes a baby or infant, whether gently or violently, causing significant brain damage. SBS has been associated with infantile death and numerous forms of developmental delays for those who survive (Kemp & Coles, 2003). The most common event leading up to the incident of shaking is extreme crying during which the baby cannot be comforted (Isser & Schwartz, 2006; Lancon, Haines, & Parent, 1998). Miehl (2005) reported that infants spend up to 20% of their waking time crying and that shaking may be directly related to the amount of frustration felt by parents while the baby is crying. Babies' heads make up about 10% of their total volume and weight, and the muscles that hold the head are extremely weak. Therefore, even a short or relatively gentle episode of shaking can cause trauma in the brain. However, how to diagnose this form of abuse is not always clear, and there is debate over the presenting symptoms of SBS.

Although many educators work outside the purview of direct infant care, compelling evidence suggests that primary prevention efforts enacted by school professionals with at-risk populations can successfully prevent SBS, thereby saving lives and preventing severe physiological and psychological symptoms. In addition to conducting primary prevention, school personnel can also play a role in identifying ongoing occurrences of SBS to prevent future incidents. It is important for school professionals to be aware of the physical symptoms of SBS, such as retinal hemorrhaging, as well as related at-risk factors to make informed decisions regarding child abuse reporting and intervention strategies.

Prevalence and Risk Factors for Shaken Baby Syndrome

It is difficult to determine the prevalence rates of SBS because identifying and diagnosing cases is challenging (Gutierrez, Clements, & Averill, 2004; Miehl, 2005). Data from the American Academy of Pediatrics (AAP)

Committee on Child Abuse and Neglect (2001) indicates that SBS is the leading cause of traumatic death and of child abuse-related deaths for infants. Typically, victims of SBS are children under 1 year of age (Ennis & Henry, 2004; Lancon et al., 1998). As a child gets older, increasing strength and weight makes older children more difficult to shake, reducing the incidence of SBS (Riffenburgh & Sathyavagiswaran, 1991b). The research reveals some conflicting information regarding the gender of the abuser, with some studies suggesting that men are more often perpetrators, while others suggesting that women more often abuse children in this way (Ennis & Henry). Males are more likely to be victims of SBS than are females, and 90% of the perpetrators of abuse of male infants are male themselves (Lancon et al.). When the perpetrator is a female, it is often a babysitter (Lancon et al.). Kivlin (2001) reported that 1,800 children suffer from SBS annually in the United States and that, of these, one third sustain fatal injuries. She also reported that several episodes of shaking often occur before the infant dies, so early detection of the subtle signs of shaking is vital in saving the child's life.

Some child factors have been identified as increasing the risk of shaking as well. Those children who were the result of an unwanted pregnancy, those who have disabilities or physical features perceived as negative by the caregivers, and those who cry inconsolably are more likely to be subject to abuse (Ennis & Henry, 2004). Meihl (2005) identified the following risk factors for SBS abusers: young parental age, unstable family environment, low socioeconomic status, infant prematurity or disability, unrealistic child-rearing expectations, rigid attitudes, parental impulsivity, depression, isolation, and negative experiences with his or her own childhood (p. 112). Kapoor et al. (1997) stated that some risk factors for SBS include "previous involvement with Child Protective Services, a history of spousal abuse, single parent families, parents who are younger than 18, parental drug and alcohol use, low socioeconomic status, or parental history of child abuse or neglect" (p. 184). However, not all researchers agree with these risk factors (Ennis & Henry). At a conference on shaken baby syndrome, researchers reported that SBS is not highly correlated to socioeconomic status, ethnicity, or parental age or level of education (Lancon et al., 1998). Ennis and Henry suggested that a powerful predictor of SBS is whether abuse has occurred previously.

Clinical Presentation of Shaken Baby Syndrome

Shaken babies often do not show the typical signs of abuse, which causes difficulty in detection (Kivlin, 2001; McCabe & Donahue, 2000; Riffenburgh & Sathyavagiswaran, 1991a). Symptoms of SBS may be internal, including subdural hemorrhages and retinal hemorrhages. The presenting signs of a baby who has suffered from SBS may include failure to thrive, diarrhea, poor feeding, irritability, hypothermia, lethargy, listlessness, apnea, vomiting, seizures, hemiplegia, upper respiratory infection, coma, and bulging anterior fontanels (i.e., the membrane-covered spaces between bones at the front of the child's skull; Hennes, Kini, & Palusci, 2001). Some of these symptoms are part of common childhood illnesses, which complicates the diagnosis of SBS. It is important that physicians are vigilant when the presenting symptoms are inconsistent with the physical findings of the child's examination (Hennes et al.). Wheeler (2003) suggested that rib fractures in babies are indicative of abuse. Miehl (2005) also identified bruises, rib fractures, long-bone fractures, and abdominal injuries as being associated with shaking trauma. Despite possible outward physical signs of abuse, SBS is often overlooked because diagnostic signs are subtle (Gutierrez et al., 2004).

Research is lacking regarding the long-term effects of survivors of SBS (Karandikar, Coles, Jayawant, & Kemp, 2004). However, longitudinal research that follows up with victims of SBS indicates that epilepsy, vision loss, and intellectual disabilities are common (Riffenburgh & Sathyavagiswaran, 1991b). Neurological complications affect as many as 57% of those who survive SBS (Hennes et al., 2001). Other difficulties may include cerebral palsy, sucking/swallowing disorders, developmental disabilities, autism, cognitive impairments, behavioral problems, deafness, paralysis, and permanent brain damage and/or vegetative states (Brooks & Weathers, 2001; Gutierrez et al., 2004).

Karandikar et al. (2004) reported on a study on 65 children under the age of 2 years who received treatment for nonaccidental head injuries, including retinal hemorrhages. Of these children, 3 were in a persistent vegetative state, 11 were "severely disabled," and 6 were "moderately disabled." Twenty-five children had "good outcomes," although the authors noted that those who were described as having good outcomes should be monitored through at least primary school to identify learning problems, behavioral problems, or special education needs that might arise later. These authors indicated that it is important to monitor carefully children who have experienced nonaccidental head injuries to insure that they receive the care they need regarding their clinical status, cognitive functioning, and educational and social needs and to provide early intervention to decrease the impact of their injuries.

Retinal Hemorrhages as Diagnostic Criteria for SBS

Unexplained and extensive retinal hemorrhages in infants are almost always diagnostic of SBS (McCabe & Donahue, 2000). Retinal hemorrhage is one of the most common findings in children who suffer from SBS (Riffenburgh & Sathyavagiswaran, 1991a), occurring in 50% to 100% of SBS victims (Kivlin, 2001; Togioka et al., 2009). Some researchers argue that the use of retinal hemorrhages is controversial in the diagnosis of SBS (Miehl, 2005). However, other researchers counter that large retinal hemorrhages are unusual in other forms of head traumas (Keenan & Runyan, 2001).

A meta-analysis of 66 published research studies examining retinal hemorrhages and SBS was recently conducted (Togioka et al., 2009). Researchers found that retinal hemorrhaging occurred bilaterally 62% to 100% of the time in confirmed SBS patients. The most common pattern observed in the retina was flame-shaped hemorrhages. The incidence of retinal hemorrhages from other forms of trauma, such as convulsions, chest compressions, persistent coughing, and forceful vomiting, were almost nonexistent. The authors stated that child abuse should be highly suspect in young children with retinal hemorrhaging and that ophthalmologic examination in suspected cases can provide essential diagnostic confirmation of SBS.

Researchers have found that children with more severe hemorrhages are more likely to experience greater neurological difficulties (Wilkinson, Han, Rappley, and Owings, 1989). Computed tomographic (CT) scans and dilated retinal examination can be performed by an ophthalmologist to rule out or diagnose SBS (Dorfman & Paradise, 1995; McCabe & Donahue, 2000). Other researchers have strongly suggested that any child who dies without obvious causes should have autopsies that included an eye exam (Riffenburgh & Sathyavagiswaran, 1991b). The American Academy of Pediatrics recommends including other signs of physical abuse, such as blunt impact, spinal cord injury, and hypoxic ischemic injury, in addition to SBS and using a broader term, such as *abusive head trauma*, to describe injury inflicted to the head of infants (Christian, Block, & American Academy of Pediatrics Committee on Child Abuse and Neglect, 2009).

Differential Diagnosis

A review of the literature on SBS indicates that the lack of specific diagnostic tools and inadequate qualifications of examiners has led to problematic differential diagnoses (Isser & Schwartz, 2006). Difficulties other than abuse that can cause ocular trauma need to be ruled out. For instance, retinal hemorrhages can result from accidental head trauma, seizures, and cardiopulmonary resuscitation (McCabe & Donahue, 2000). Additionally, intracranial hemorrhaging and/or brain damage can be caused by premature birth, apnea, aneurysms, brittle-bone disease, or hydrocephalus (Isser & Schwartz). It is important to complete a careful history and physical examination to determine the reason for the hemorrhages. Retinal hemorrhages can occur during the birth process, but after the neonatal period, these hemorrhages are rare. Therefore, some researchers believe retinal hemorrhages should be considered a sign of child abuse (Togioka et al., 2009; Wheeler, 2003).

Those who shake a baby often deny their involvement in the child's injury and report that accidents are to blame for the child's injuries. Studies have shown that the type of brain injury that occurs would require a fall of at least 4 to 5 feet onto a hard surface (Lancon et al., 1998). Generally, falls from beds do not result in serious brain injuries (Miehl, 2005; Wheeler, 2003). However, the most common explanation given by caregivers is that the child fell out of a bed with a height of 2 to 3 feet.

Prevention and Intervention

Research suggests that public awareness of the dangers of shaking a baby has increased over the past decade. Therefore, an important role of prevention programs is to reintroduce the information to parents at critical times (Dias et al., 2005). Fostering an improved understanding of the impact of shaking a baby leads to a lessening of the behavior (Gutierrez et al., 2004). Education programs aimed at informing parents or parents-to-be about the dangers of shaking a baby are effective at decreasing this form of abuse.

According to Dias and colleagues (2005), 93% of parents in their study were already familiar with the dangers of shaking an infant. The authors stated that adults learn best when information is practical and well aligned with their current life circumstances. The most appropriate time to provide a primary prevention program is at the hospital when a baby is born. Pantrini (2002) urged that prevention of SBS must include the message that asking for and seeking help is not a sign of failure but rather is an act of responsible parenting.

Research regarding the effectiveness of primary and secondary prevention programs in reducing the incidence of SBS is limited (Hennes et al., 2001). *Primary prevention* refers to intervention with the general public, before any risk factors are identified. *Secondary prevention* is intervention aimed at families at high risk for or with a history of engaging in abusive behaviors. Primary prevention efforts that target SBS have increased, but evaluation of the effectiveness of these programs is in its infancy. Secondary prevention efforts targeting populations at risk have not been shown to be effective because of the many co-occurring risk factors, such as income, gender, and relationship between victim and perpetrator.

Nagler (2002) indicated that providing education and teaching healthy coping strategies is important in the prevention of SBS. The most effective form of prevention is secondary prevention (Davies & Garwood, 2001). Research is increasingly identifying those populations with specific risk or protective factors to facilitate more targeted interventions.

Showers (2001) indicated that one potential challenge to preventing SBS is the message that there are times when it is appropriate, even medically necessary, to shake an infant. Showers reported that cardiopulmonary resuscitation (CPR) instructions for infants include the instruction to "shake" when an infant is not breathing and that parents have been advised to shake an infant with apnea. The use of these instructions has decreased recently, but further public safety advisories are necessary.

IMPLICATIONS FOR EDUCATORS

Because many cases result in death, SBS may not seem like an issue that is directly related to the work of school professionals. However, victims of abuse might recover physically but still experience a variety of psychological difficulties, including low academic achievement, shyness, low self-esteem, and more acting-out behavior (Chiocca, 1995). Children who experience serious traumatic brain injury before age 6 progress more slowly and experience more difficulty gaining new skills than their peers (Keenan & Runyan, 2001). Survivors of SBS experience complications such as visual impairments, motor impairments, seizures, and developmental delays. Long-term effects of SBS may require continued medical care, physical therapy, occupational therapy, speech/language therapy, and educational interventions (Dias et al., 2005). Many cases of SBS go unnoticed, and special educators may encounter students who unknowingly have been victims of SBS. Therefore, interventions with these students may resemble interventions with students who experience difficulty learning, attending, remembering, and mastering language.

SBS-related services (including special education, foster care placement, and child protective services) are conservatively estimated to cost $5 million to $10 million annually (Hennes et al., 2001). Many follow-up services, including speech/language, vision, physical, or occupational therapies, may be required to address a variety of difficulties. Additionally, it may be necessary to gain the assistance of feeding specialists or behavioral specialists (Gutierrez et al., 2004). Significant speech problems and learning disabilities might not appear in affected children until several years after the traumatic event (Gedieit, 2001).

Several instructional and compensatory strategies may be useful for students who have been victims of shaking. To address visual-perceptual issues, students may benefit from use of large-print books, books on tape, and longer viewing times or repeat viewings when using visual materials. Auditory processing may also be difficult for a student who has experienced a brain injury from shaking. Some instructional strategies to address auditory processing concerns can include limiting the amount of information presented verbally, providing repetition, using concrete terms, allowing for preferential seating, and teaching the student to self-advocate and ask questions when information is unclear.

It is important to match students' strengths to their needs, particularly with students who have brain injuries. If a student has poor vision but is a strong auditory learner, for example, information should be presented verbally or via a multisensory approach. Additionally, it may be useful to limit the amount of new information presented at one time and to tie new learning to rote, well-habitualized skills. Explicit instruction in note taking and using a planner/datebook may be helpful with students who suffer from SBS, as memory may be negatively affected. Other compensatory strategies for memory difficulties include chunking, mnemonic devices, and rehearsal/repetition. Problem solving can also be negatively impacted by brain injuries caused by shaking. Strategies for improving problem-solving skills include providing the student with a problem-solving guide or flow chart to help the child learn the steps in solving a problem, using group discussions to brainstorm solutions to problems and to evaluate the outcomes, and providing feedback related to student choices (State Education Department, USNY, 2002).

A major risk factor for SBS is parents having developmentally inappropriate expectations of a child (Butler, 1995). One of the primary reasons parents have unrealistic expectations is a lack of knowledge about developmentally appropriate behaviors (Chiocca, 1995). School psychologists and educators are instrumental in providing community education programs that outline development milestones, methods to nurture children, and ways to cope with stress and frustration and prevent child abuse. This is particularly important for parents still in high school, as becoming a parent at a young age is a significant risk factor for perpetrating child abuse (Kruger, 1997; Swenson & Levitt, 1997). Additionally, since babysitters sometimes abuse the children in their care, they should be trained in ways to deal with a crying or colicky baby.

Swenson and Levitt (1997) provided several suggestions for physicians to be more involved with the prevention of SBS. Many of these suggestions can be extended to the educator's role as well. For instance, they recommended that professionals become aware of community resources, such as parent support groups and parenting classes. School psychologists, teachers, social workers, and counselors can refer families to agencies that can help them cope with the stressors of having a newborn and provide them with developmental information about their babies. Additionally, the authors recommended providing information about SBS for parents to take home. Although the educator's focus is typically on school-aged children, parents often have other children at home, and providing this information can be helpful in preventing SBS and ensuring the safety of all children. The authors also noted that it is important to validate parents' concerns and frustrations about having a baby in the home. Educators can provide empathetic support and suggestions for parents who report they are experiencing high levels of stress in the home.

Conclusion

Showers (2001) argued that the responsibility of educating people about SBS falls on all professionals who work with parents or children. She stated that school professionals are in a position where they can provide education in a brief session to parents, as well as to adolescent students who might become babysitters or parents. Research on the effects of preventing SBS from a psychoeducational perspective is lacking (Kruger, 1997). Educators and other professionals could assist in adding to the research base and helping to elucidate the physical, psychological, and educational ramifications of SBS.

It is important that school employees consider their ethical and legal requirements to report suspected cases of abuse. When young children present with unexplained symptoms that may be associated with SBS, it is important to gather all supporting information and, if indicated, make referrals for further investigation. This action is not only prudent and lawful but could ultimately save a child's life.

EDUCATIONAL STRATEGIES

- Present information using a multisensory approach to maximize the amount of information learned.
- Use chunking, mnemonic devices, and rehearsal/repetition to target memory weaknesses.
- To address poor problem solving, teach explicit problem-solving strategies. A guide or flow chart may help students to learn problem-solving steps, and group brainstorming may be helpful. Teach students to evaluate the possible outcomes of their choices.
- Teach students to self-monitor their attending skills and provide them with signals to redirect their attention. Preferential seating and/or 1:1 instruction may be necessary.
- Direct prevention and education efforts at parents who seem overwhelmed with their newborns, as well as at adolescents who are pregnant, fathers-to-be, or babysitters. These efforts can include training in child care, child development, and methods to sooth and nurture an infant and instructions on how to access community services when caregivers feel overwhelmed.

DISCUSSION QUESTIONS

1. What is the role of medical/health professionals in educating expecting parents about stress associated with crying babies?
2. What responsibilities do school personnel have in educating parents, children, and/or adolescents about shaken baby syndrome?
3. What steps should an early childhood educator or child care provider take when SBS is suspected?

4. Should expectant parents meeting certain risk conditions be targeted for SBS prevention training? If so, what risk conditions would meet criteria for inclusion?

RESEARCH SUMMARY

- Infants spend up to 20% of their waking time crying, and shaking may be directly related to the amount of frustration felt by parents while the baby is crying.
- The presenting signs of a baby who has suffered from SBS may include failure to thrive, diarrhea, poor feeding, irritability, hypothermia, lethargy, listlessness, apnea, vomiting, seizures, hemiplegia (i.e., paralysis of right or left side of the body), upper respiratory infection, coma, and bulging anterior fontanels.
- Unexplained and extensive retinal hemorrhages in infants are almost diagnostic of SBS, occurring in 50% to 100% of SBS victims. The retinal hemorrhaging often occurs in a distinctive flame shape pattern.
- Child abuse should be strongly suspected in young children with retinal hemorrhaging, and ophthalmologic examination in suspected cases can provide essential diagnostic confirmation that SBS has occurred.
- It is important for school personnel to identify learning problems, behavioral problems, or special education needs that may arise for survivors of SBS.
- Research is limited on survivors of SBS; however, school personnel may work with survivors without knowing it. Symptoms of SBS survival may present under another disorder, such as traumatic brain injury, ADHD, learning disabilities, blindness, and so on.

RESOURCES

The National Center of Shaken Baby Syndrome Web site (www.dontshake .org) provides basic information regarding prevention, coping with crying, signs/symptoms of shaking, what to do if you suspect your child has been shaken, and stories of victims and survivors. *The Period of PURPLE Crying*, an evidence-based SBS prevention program that includes a booklet and DVD, can be purchased through the Web site.

Additionally, the New York State Department of Health Web site (www.health.state.ny.us/nysdoh/consumer/sbs) offers information on introducing an infant to siblings along with tips on how parents can take care of themselves and calm an inconsolable infant. A chart shows what is developmentally appropriate for infants up to age 3. This Web site offers brochures on SBS in English, French, Spanish, Russian, and Chinese.

The following Web sites provide information on basic developmental milestones to help parents and caregivers understand what is typically expected from a baby at certain ages:

Child Development Guide: www.child-development-guide.com/child-development-milestone.html

WebMD ("Is Your Baby on Track?"): www.webmd.com/parenting/guide/is-your-baby-on-track

HANDOUT

PREVENTING SHAKEN BABY SYNDROME

Shaken baby syndrome (SBS) has received increased media attention in recent years. Many people assume it is well known that shaking a child is dangerous and can cause brain damage, blindness, or death. However, cases of SBS still occur today in alarming numbers.

Information for Caregivers

- Babies can spend up to 20% of their waking time crying (Miehl, 2005). That's a lot! It can be frustrating to hear a baby cry, and especially frustrating when nothing seems to help. Pay close attention to your own stress during this time.
- Learn how to decrease your own stress levels. Hearing a baby cry inconsolably can be very frustrating. Try several different methods of calming the baby, including feeding, rocking, checking the diaper, singing or talking to the baby, going for a walk or ride, or using a baby swing. If nothing works, find another adult to help and take a break! You need to take care of yourself before you can take care of a baby.
- Older children in the family also need to be aware of how to handle the infant, including how to hold a baby properly and soothe it. An older sibling can also be frustrated by inconsolable crying and may react by shaking the infant if he or she is not taught how to relate to an infant properly. The same is true for inexperienced babysitters.
- Know when to seek help. Asking for help from professionals is not a sign of weakness or an indicator of being ill-prepared to be a parent or babysitter. Rather, it shows that you want the best for the baby and are willing to seek help to do so.
- Educate yourself and other people taking care of the child. Several prevention programs are offered at hospitals at the time of a birth. Ask to be enrolled in a program or to receive information when you are at the hospital. When choosing someone to look after the infant, ask candidates about their experience with crying and how they will handle it. Provide your caregiver with information on the dangers of shaking.

Information for Babysitters

- When babysitting, ask what behaviors you should expect and what the parents do to help the baby when he or she is crying. For instance, it might be helpful to know that babies do not typically sit up by themselves until around 4 months or crawl until 6 months. If you know what to expect, you won't be surprised when the baby doesn't do something.
- If you find yourself in a situation with an infant that you can't handle, get help. Try to find the parents or an adult to help you manage the situation.
- Talk to the parents if caring for a young child is too stressful for you. They will be able to find another babysitter, and they will appreciate your self-awareness and your commitment to keeping their child safe.
- Information on shaken baby syndrome is not always included in babysitter training programs. Seek out this information and training on your own, if necessary.

6

Assessment and Intervention for Sleep Problems*

Joseph A. Buckhalt and Mona El-Sheikh

Matt is a 7-year-old boy who lives with his mother, Eloise M.; an older sister (9 years old); and an older half-brother (16 years old) in a small, two-bedroom, single-family home. Ms. M. is employed as a school bus driver. Other than having had tubes implanted for ear infections in infancy, Matt has an unremarkable medical history, but he has frequent colds. His height is within the average range, and his weight is above average, according to standard growth charts. He attended a day care center from age 3 to 5, with no problems reported. Periodic problems in attention and occasional noncompliance were reported by teachers in kindergarten and first grade.

Matt's second-grade teacher contacted the school psychologist in October after learning that he was taking 18 mg of methylphenidate (Concerta) daily. The teacher was aware that Concerta is a medication prescribed for children with ADHD and said that while he did have some attention problems, they were no worse than those of several others in the class. Matt had not been referred for school assessment.

Matt was assessed by the school psychologist, who conducted a classroom observation, parent and child clinical interview, Child Behavior Checklist, Revised Children's Manifest Anxiety Scale, Five-Factor Personality Inventory for Children, Pediatric Sleep Questionnaire (PSQ), sleep diary, and 1 week of actigraphy.

Matt was observed in the classroom on two occasions for 40-minute periods, once during the morning (8:30–9:10 a.m.) and once during the afternoon (1:10–1:50 p.m.). Interval recording indicated that he was on-task 62% during the morning and 53% during the afternoon observation. A target comparison

*Adapted from Buckhalt, J. A., Wolfson, A., & El-Sheikh, M. (2007). Children's sleep, academic performance, and school behavior. *Communiqué, 35*(8), 40–43. Copyright by the National Association of School Psychologists, Bethesda, MD. Use is by permission of the publisher. www.nasponline.org

child had on-task percentages of 78% in the morning and 73% in the afternoon. Matt's mother reported that he is irritable and noncompliant after school and during early evening hours, but he usually settles down after dinner. She also said that Matt is much more active than her other two children have been and that her pediatrician had suggested a trial of methylphenidate.

The PSQ showed elevated scores for Excessive Daytime Sleepiness and Inattentive/Hyperactive Behavior. Interviews with Matt and his mother revealed that Matt shares a room with his older brother, who typically stays up watching TV in his room until 11:00 p.m. on school nights. Matt has to go to bed by 10:00 p.m., and the brother is supposed to turn down the sound at that time. Matt's mother must leave home at 5:30 a.m. for work, so his older siblings are responsible for making sure that he gets up, gets dressed, eats breakfast, has school materials ready, and is ready for the bus, which arrives at 7:00 a.m. He has football practice one afternoon a week and an early evening game once a week. Results from 1 week of actigraphy and a sleep diary indicated that Matt's time of sleep onset averaged 10:47 p.m. on school nights and 11:32 p.m. on weekends. Wake time averages were 6:22 a.m. on school mornings and 8:17 a.m. on weekends. Average sleep times were 7 hr 33 min school nights and 8 hr 45 min on weekends. Sleep onset times varied considerably from night to night. Of the time spent in bed, Matt was asleep only 64% of the time, with frequent awakenings during most nights.

Following assessment, Matt and his mother met with the school psychologist for an instructional session with PowerPoint slides on the importance of sleep and recommendations for sleep hygiene. A comprehensive 6-week intervention plan was prepared, which included self- and parent-monitored bedtime; elimination of caffeinated drinks on school afternoons and evenings; and institution of a pre-bedtime routine that included no television, stimulating activities, or snacking 2 hours before bedtime. A behavioral contract was written to encourage compliance. For the 1st week, the school psychologist called every evening to remind the family about routines and to collect information from a sleep diary. Phone prompts were faded gradually such that by the end of the intervention, one call a week was made. The school psychologist consulted with Matt's teacher, and an intervention was implemented consisting of daily on-task charts and reinforcements for attending to instructions and staying on-task.

At the end of intervention, 1 week of actigraphy showed that Matt was sleeping 88% of the time he spent in bed. Sleep times on school nights increased to 8 hr 7 min, and there was less variability in sleep onset times and fewer awakenings during the night. Improvement was also seen in PSQ scores. Charts of on-task behavior showed improvement over the 6 weeks that was satisfactory to the teacher.

INTRODUCTION

Substantial research has shown relations between poor sleep and problematic functioning in children and adolescents. Children with sleep disorders and healthy children who have problems with sleep often have a wide range of problems, including mood disturbances, behavior problems, and poor performance on cognitive and academic tasks (Sadeh, 2007). Further, sleep disturbance is associated with numerous psychiatric disorders and physical health problems in children as well as adults.

Although the majority of studies have been of children who have clinical conditions, relations between sleep and many behaviors in typically developing, healthy children are receiving increased attention. More than two dozen studies have related sleep problems to cognitive and academic performance measures, including vigilance and attention, working memory, executive functioning, individual and group intelligence and performance on achievement tests, and school grades (Buckhalt, Wolfson, & El-Sheikh, 2009). In addition, a number of experimental studies have demonstrated causal connections between sleep loss and impaired cognitive performance (e.g., Sadeh, Gruber, & Raviv, 2003). These results are particularly troubling in view of evidence that U.S. children and adolescents (along with adults) are generally sleeping less than what is recommended for optimal functioning (National Sleep Foundation, 2004), as well as the frequent and alarming reports of what is characterized as underachievement on standardized tests of academic performance (U.S. Department of Education, 2008).

BACKGROUND

Shortened sleep time, erratic sleep/wake schedules, late bedtimes and rise times, and poor sleep quality are associated with poorer school performance (Sadeh, 2007). School performance outcomes have been measured by teacher ratings and grades, individual and group achievement tests, specialized tests of cognitive functioning, and standardized batteries of intelligence. For example, poorer sleep has been associated with poorer scores on the Reading, Mathematics, and Language scores of the Stanford Achievement Test (Buckhalt, El-Sheikh, Keller, & Kelly, 2009). Sleep loss causes dysfunction in the prefrontal lobes of the brain with corresponding inefficiency in working memory and executive processes. Although the preponderance of the literature consists of correlational studies, where cause and effect cannot be proved, many experimental studies with adults and the few with children have shown that less sleep and poor sleep causes the problems (Sadeh et al., 2003).

Other studies have compared sleep/wake patterns and academic performance for earlier- versus later-starting middle or high schools or for students who do their best work in the morning versus those who function best in the afternoon/evening. The studies suggest that self-reported eveningness, delayed sleep schedules, and early school start times are associated with daytime sleepiness, dozing in class, attention difficulties, and poorer academic performance (Wolfson, Spaulding, Dandrow, & Baroni, 2007).

Diagnostic Considerations for Sleep Disorders

Sleep of children with clinically diagnosed conditions has been studied extensively. First, there are children who have diagnosed sleep disorders. These disorders are classified in two diagnostic systems, the *International Classification of Sleep Disorders* (*ICSD-2*; AASM, 2005), and the *Diagnostic and Statistical Manual of Mental Disorders*, text revision (*DSM-IV-TR*, APA, 2000). Children with sleep disorders have been found to have problems in numerous cognitive, behavioral, emotional, and health domains, and these problems are related to academic performance and behavior at home and school (Halbower & Mahone, 2006).

Another category of clinical conditions includes children whose primary diagnosis is not a sleep disorder but another clinical condition. Sleep problems in children and adolescents with ADHD have been reported, and some portion of children with ADHD may have undiagnosed sleep disorders (Cohen-Zion & Ancoli-Israel, 2004). Depression and bipolar disorder are also associated with sleep disorders (Ivanenko, Crabtree, & Gozal, 2005). Children with intellectual disabilities, autism spectrum disorders, and other developmental disorders experience a high rate of sleep problems (Stores & Wiggs, 2001). For autism, between 44% and 83% of children report some type and degree of problem with sleep (Williams, Sears, & Allard, 2004). Similarly high rates, from 34% to 80%, have been reported for children with intellectual disabilities (Richdale, Francis, Gavidia-Payne, & Cotton, 2000). Children with epilepsy also have more sleep disorders than healthy children (Cortesi, Giannotti, & Ottaviano, 1999).

Children who are experiencing acute or chronic stressors typically manifest sleep problems that may be transient but may also become long-lasting. Sleep problems are common among abused children, and environmental stressors, such as those associated with wars, terrorist attacks, and natural disasters, precipitate sleep disturbance. Even stressors associated with normative levels of marital conflict and emotional insecurity have been related to sleep problems.

Sleep and Heath Correlates

One of the most prevalent medical disorders affecting children is asthma. Good breathing is necessary for quality sleep, and children with asthma have been shown to have problems falling asleep, difficulty staying asleep, and poor sleep quality. These problems, in turn, are related to fatigue, difficulty in concentrating, and irritability (Desager, Nelen, Weyler, & De Backer, 2004).

Another serious health concern is overweight and obesity, for which rates in the United States are rising at an alarming rate. These children have high rates of sleep problems (Redline et al., 1999), partly due to airway obstruction associated with higher body mass but also due to the nighttime regulation of hormones controlling appetite (Amin & Daniels, 2002). Obesity and asthma co-occur in many children, and sleep problems may add to difficulties these children experience at school. Even though obesity affects children of all social classes, the highest rates occur among those with the lowest incomes.

Differences in academic achievement by race and socioeconomic status (SES) groups may be explained partially by the fact that poor sleep can compromise cognitive performance and school achievement (Buckhalt, El-Sheikh, et al., 2009). In those studies, African-American and European-American children and those from lower and higher SES homes had similar scores on ability and achievement tests when they had good sleep quality and less variability in sleep, but when sleep was disrupted, lower-SES and African-American children had poorer performance.

Adolescent Sleep Patterns

Emotional dysregulation and poor school performance have been associated with insufficient sleep in adolescence (Dahl & Lewin, 2002). The biological need for sleep (about 9 hr) does not change from ages 10 to 17 (Carskadon & Acebo, 2002). Yet the timing of sleep changes as children enter and pass through adolescence; they tend to stay up later in the evening and need to sleep later in the morning. This shift in sleep has a biological component linked to melatonin levels, which peak later in the evening in comparison to those of younger children and adults. The delayed sleep pattern is most obvious on weekends, whereas sleep schedules are largely determined on weekdays by school start-time schedules. As a result, when adolescents need to rise earlier than their natural wake time to get ready for school, but need more sleep, they often experience excessive daytime sleepiness. Survey results consistently indicate that middle and high school students who start school at 7:15 a.m. or earlier have less sleep on school nights in comparison to students at later starting schools (Wolfson et al., 2007). Many school districts have considered adolescent sleep needs and shifted to later high school start times.

Assessing Sleep Problems

Educators and clinicians have a number of ways to assess sleep in diagnosing and treating sleep problems. Self-report questionnaires give a broad overview of a child's sleep/wake patterns. The Pediatric Sleep Questionnaire (PSQ; Chervin, Hedger, Dillon, & Pituch, 2000) and the Children's Sleep Habits Questionnaire (CSHQ; Owens, Spirito, & McGuinn, 2000) are useful for assessing common sleep disorders and sleep-related problems. The School Sleep Habits Survey (SHS; Wolfson et al., 2003) asks older children and adolescents about their sleep patterns, daytime sleepiness, and sleep/wake behavior problems in the last 2 weeks. The BEARS is a brief screening instrument designed for pediatricians to use when interviewing parents and children (ages 2 to 18) as part of taking a sleep history (Owens & Dalzell, 2005). The Sleep Disorders Inventory for Students (SDIS; Luginbuehl, 2003) is a normed instrument with separate versions for children and adolescents and a Spanish-language version. All of these instruments have acceptable reliability and validity and are appropriate for screening purposes; unfortunately, none has been developed on a stratified national norming sample.

Daytime sleepiness is important to evaluate but difficult to assess with great precision. The Multiple Sleep Latency Test (MSLT), developed for use with both adults and children (Carskadon et al., 1986), is conducted during the day in a laboratory, where the person lies in a darkened bedroom and is encouraged to go to sleep. After a polysomnogram (PSG) determines that sleep is present for a predetermined period, the person is awakened. Then the procedure is repeated at several intervals during the day. The time it takes the person to fall asleep is the measure of sleepiness, with greater sleepiness operationally defined as *rapid sleep onset*. Given the practical limitations of MSLT, the primary means of measuring sleepiness has been with self-report scales. Many of the self-report instruments mentioned above have an item or short scale addressing sleepiness, and the Pediatric Daytime Sleepiness Scale (PDSS; Drake et al., 2003), a scale developed solely for measuring sleepiness, is a good choice for school-based screening. Relationships between high PDSS scores were found with absenteeism, low achievement, low school enjoyment, low total sleep time, and high rates of illness. In addition to these measures, sleepiness may also be inferred when children sleep substantially more on weekends than school days, the assumption being that weekends allow for paying back sleep "debt."

IMPLICATIONS FOR EDUCATORS

- Teachers should become familiar with the signs of sleepiness in children and refer those children to school psychologists and counselors. Sleep problems should be ruled out before assuming that children have learning and/or behavior problems.
- Children who have serious learning and/or behavior problems may also have sleep problems. Assessment and interventions to improve sleep should be considered for comprehensive evaluation and treatment plans.
- Parents often need help finding appropriate health care services to support sleep and address sleep-related problems. Physicians or psychologists in the community may be able to help with some kinds of problems, whereas more serious problems (e.g., sleep apnea) should be referred to sleep medicine specialists. Many hospitals have sleep centers, but fewer have pediatric sleep specialists.

EDUCATIONAL STRATEGIES

- When students are suspected of getting insufficient sleep, formal and informal assessment of sleep should be done.
- Based on the sleep assessment, consultation and education should be implemented with parents to improve sleep. Specific strategies include use of sleep diaries and improvement of the social and physical environment related to good sleep (see "Tips for Parents" in the handout at the end of this chapter).
- Children whose sleep cannot be improved through consultation with parents should be seen by school counselors or psychologists, who can in some cases implement cognitive-behavior therapy methods.
- Because many children may be sleepy both early and late in the school day, the timing of classroom tests and group-administered achievement tests should be considered.
- In the weeks preceding high-stakes testing, schoolwide efforts should be made to have students get adequate sleep.
- Similar to what is done for nutrition, hygiene, and exercise, formal and informal health education should emphasize the benefits of good sleep and the risks associated with poor sleep.

- Educators can also speak to students from time to time about good sleep habits. When traumatic events disturbing to children occur, interventions to help with sleep problems should be included in crisis management.
- Districtwide policies that may affect students' sleep and sleepiness should be discussed.

DISCUSSION QUESTIONS

1. To what extent do you believe school-related problems of children and adolescents are caused by, or related to, sleep problems?

2. What prevention and intervention sleep programs do you think are justified for children? Do you think those programs should be based in schools, in pediatric clinics, in hospitals, or elsewhere?

3. Ask yourself: Has my performance in school or work ever been adversely affected by lack of sleep or poor sleep? Discuss with others the ways in which sleep has affected your performance.

4. Do you consider your sleep to be of sufficient length and quality? Do you consider the sleep of your friends and family to be sufficient?

5. Given the demands and opportunities of contemporary life, how can sufficient sleep be made a bigger priority?

RESEARCH SUMMARY

- Children who have diagnosed sleep disorders have been shown to have problems in learning and behavior.
- Likewise, a great many children who have school-identified learning and behavior disorders have problems sleeping.
- Sleep in sufficient quantity and quality is necessary for all developing children in multiple domains, including physical growth, healthy immune functioning, hormonal regulation, learning, and emotional control.
- Health problems related to insufficient or problem sleep patterns include asthma and overweight/obesity, for which rates in the United States are rising at an alarming rate. Obesity and asthma co-occur in many children, and sleep problems may add to the difficulties these children experience at school. Even though obesity affects children of all social classes, the highest rates occur among those with the lowest income.
- Schools have not been a setting where sleep is assessed or related to children's problems.
- Emotional dysregulation and poor school performance have been associated with insufficient sleep in adolescence. Many school districts have considered adolescent sleep needs and shifted to later high school start times.

RESOURCES

Donaldson, D. L., & Owens, J. A. (2006). Sleep and sleep problems. In G. G. Bear & K. M. Minke (Eds.), *Children's needs III: Development, prevention, and intervention* (pp. 1025–1039). Bethesda, MD: National Association of School Psychologists.

Ivanenko, A. (Ed.). (2008). *Sleep and psychiatric disorders in children and adolescents.* New York: Informa Healthcare.

Mindell, J. A. (2005). *Sleeping through the night: How infants, toddlers, and their parents can get a good night's sleep.* New York: HarperCollins.

National Institutes of Health (NIH) & National Heart, Lung, and Blood Institute (NHLBI). (2003). *Sleep, sleep disorders, and biological rhythms: NIH curriculum supplement series—Grades 9–12.* Colorado Springs, CO: BSCS. Retrieved September 19, 2009, from http://science.education.nih.gov/supplements/nih3/sleep/default.htm

Owens, J. A., & Mindell, J. A. (2005). *Take charge of your child's sleep: The all-in-one resource for solving sleep problems in kids and teens.* New York: Marlowe.

The following Web sites contain information about healthful sleep and sleep disorders:

American Academy of Sleep Medicine: www.sleepeducation.com; www.sleepcenters.org (to locate a sleep diagnosis and treatment center near you)

National Sleep Foundation: www.sleepfoundation.org

Sleep for Kids: www.sleepforkids.org

H A N D O U T

SLEEP DISORDERS

Basic Facts

- Children 5 to 12 years old need 10 to 11 hours of sleep; teenagers need 8½ to 10 hours.
- Puberty brings hormonal changes that make it difficult to fall asleep early in the evening. These biological changes, combined with social pressures that support teens staying up later, favor later morning sleep that is not compatible with early school start times.
- Sleeping well is essential for optimal learning and recall of information. Learned material is retained better if followed by quality sleep.
- Sleep loss is related to mood and behavior problems. Loss of sleep impairs the ability to regulate emotions and behavior, which, in turn, often leads to conflict with friends, teachers, and family members.
- Hormones that control appetite (e.g., leptin, ghrelin) are affected by sleep loss, and their dysregulation is thought to be the cause of the recently discovered link between poor sleep and obesity/overweight in children.
- Children who live in high-conflict homes often do not sleep well, and many of the negative outcomes these children experience are due to the combination of direct effects of stressors (e.g., anxiety; depression) and the indirect effects of inability to sleep well.

Tips for Parents

- Monitor and enforce the amount of sleep children get. Because school begins early, bedtimes must be early to allow for 9 to 11 hours of sleep. Bedtime routines should be set and closely supervised with few exceptions allowed. Ideally, bedrooms should not have telephones, computers, electronic games, and televisions, and activities near bedtime should be quiet ones.
- Late-night eating should be avoided. Caffeinated drinks should be either prohibited or limited during the day and especially during late the afternoon and evening.
- Dimmer lighting in the evening facilitates sleep, and bright light exposure, especially sunlight, in the morning helps with awakening.
- Consistency of bedtimes from night to night should be a priority. For weekend nights, bedtimes should not be much later. If children are sleeping more than 1 hour longer on weekend nights, then that is evidence that children are sleep deprived during the week and likely not performing their best.
- When possible, each child should have his or her own sleeping space. Bed sharing should be avoided. Adequate temperature and humidity control in bedrooms is required for good sleep.
- Good sleep requires good breathing. Nasal congestion due to colds and allergies should be treated with children's decongestants that do not impair sleep and with nasal dilator strips that open nasal passages. Snoring should always be taken as a sign that breathing is not good, and children who snore chronically should have a medical exam.
- Adults and older children who stay up later than younger children should keep sound and light levels down in the house.
- Parents should model good sleep habits by making their own good sleep a priority.
- Children and their parents can help track quality and quantity of sleep by keeping sleep diaries, completing sleep problems questionnaires, and monitoring napping and daytime sleepiness.
- For children suspected of having a serious sleep problem, the help of a school counselor or school psychologist should be sought. For some cases, a pediatrician or sleep medicine specialist should be consulted.

7

Cognitive Effects of Childhood Leukemia Treatments*

Paul C. McCabe

José was midway through the first grade when he developed an extended illness. After a series of medical tests, his parents were notified that José suffered from acute myelogenous leukemia. The medical team initiated a chemotherapy protocol using a strong dose of intravenous methotrexate in an effort to prevent further spreading of the cancer. The chemotherapy protocol called for three 5-day intravenous injections, ranging in duration from several hours up to 24 hours a day. José experienced significant side effects, including frequent nausea, vomiting, transient pain, hair loss, and jaundice. Because of his nausea and vomiting, José was unable to eat most solid foods, thus requiring intravenously administered nutrition. His appearance upon discharge from the hospital was remarkably different from that at admission, with a gaunt, jaundiced pallor, sunken cheeks, darkened circles around his eyes, and slowed physical movement. He went home for 2 weeks of rest and recuperation before returning to school.

(Continued)

*Adapted from Kretz, H. L., & McCabe, P. C. (2003). Childhood leukemia treatment: Cognitive outcomes. *Communiqué*, 32(3), 28–30. Copyright by the National Association of School Psychologists, Bethesda, MD. Use is by permission of the publisher. www.nasponline.org

(Continued)

Shortly after José's diagnosis, his parents contacted his teacher, Ms. Gladstein, and informed her of the diagnosis and proposed medical plan. José's parents also passed this information to the school psychologist, Mr. Walsh, who obtained parental consent to act as a liaison among the family, educational teams, and medical teams. Mr. Walsh and Ms. Gladstein stayed in contact with the medical team and the family throughout the chemotherapy treatment and subsequent home recovery. José's parents and medical team informed Mr. Walsh when they believed that José was feeling strong enough to start working on academics. A temporary home-based instructor was assigned to work with José for 2 hours a day, which was the maximum time that José could sustain attention without excessive fatigue.

José's parents and the school team decided to reintroduce José to school on a half-time basis until his strength fully recovered. A tentative plan for 1 week of half-day morning classes was developed. In preparation, Ms. Gladstein spoke to the class about José's illness and his impending return to the classroom. She encouraged the class to be supportive and optimistic. Ms. Gladstein also cautioned the class that José would look somewhat different from before and would be wearing a baseball cap. She told the class that José needed their support and any teasing would not be tolerated.

José's reintegration to the class went smoothly. The class was openly curious about his hair loss and hospital experience. José spoke about his experience and brought some hospital paraphernalia (IV tubes, tape, etc.) to describe what happened. In addition, José's parents and Ms. Gladstein participated in a planned 45-minute presentation to the entire first grade. This provided information to José's peers and teachers regarding his form of leukemia and upcoming chemotherapy treatments. Because José was expected to miss more school in the future and manifest physiological and psychological effects from the treatment, it was important to prepare his peers and teachers.

Ms. Gladstein noted that, in addition to having missed significant academic content during the year, José exhibited subtle symptoms of cognitive delay and slowing. He seemed to take much longer to read beginner passages, and he had difficulty retaining quantitative concepts in working memory long enough to complete arithmetic problems. To remedy this, Ms. Gladstein gave José a variety of manipulative materials, such as beads and blocks, to help him represent math problems without relying entirely on working memory. She also brought her concerns to the school multidisciplinary team to discuss other options for remedial support and further assessment. The additional supports that were provided helped José finish the school year with his class, and he was promoted to second grade.

INTRODUCTION

Cancer is the term used to describe a category of diseases in which cells in the body mutate and begin to multiply rapidly. Although the occurrence of cancer in children and adolescents is relatively rare in comparison to its occurrence in adults, cancer is the second leading cause of death in children age 14 and under (American Cancer Society, 2009). One particular type of cancer, leukemia, is especially prevalent among the types of cancer found in children and adolescents.

BACKGROUND

Definition of Leukemia

According to the American Cancer Society (2009), *leukemia* is a cancer of the white blood cells. This form of cancer originates in the bone marrow and can then spread to the blood, lymph nodes, central nervous system, and organs. Leukemia, when diagnosed in children, typically falls under only two of the four major categories of leukemia. Children identified as having leukemia usually have either acute lymphocytic leukemia or acute myelogenous leukemia. The first major type, acute lymphocytic leukemia, is a cancer of the lymphocyte-forming cells (which are B-cells or T-cells). This is the most common type of childhood leukemia. The second major type, acute myelogenous leukemia, is a cancer of the bone marrow cells that form granulocytes, monocytes, red blood cells, and platelets (American Cancer Society).

Overall, leukemia accounts for approximately one third of all cancers in children under the age of 15 and approximately one fourth of all cancers in those less than 20 years of age (American Cancer Society, 2009). The American Cancer Society predicted that during 2009, about 3,500 children in the United Sates would be diagnosed with leukemia. Of those 3,500 new cases, roughly 3 of 4 would be acute lymphocyte leukemia, with the majority of the remaining cases being acute myelogenous leukemia. Acute lymphocyte leukemia is most often diagnosed in early childhood, peaking between 2 and 4 years of age, while acute myelogenous cases occur throughout childhood with slight peaks before age 2 and during adolescence (American Cancer Society).

Etiology and Treatment

The exact cause of leukemia remains unknown. Effective treatments for childhood leukemia have greatly improved the survival rate of children who develop this form of cancer. According to the American Cancer Society (2009), more than 95% of children with acute lymphocytic leukemia now enter remission after 1 month of treatment. The long-term survival rate for children with leukemia is currently greater than 70% (Armstrong, Blumberg, & Toledano, 1999). Over 91% of children under 5 survive acute lymphocytic leukemia, and just over 60% of children under age 15 survive acute myelogenous leukemia (Leukemia & Lymphoma Society, 2009).

The treatment for childhood leukemia usually consists of 2 to 3 years of intense drug therapy. Children with leukemia typically receive either systemic chemotherapy, which is usually administered intravenously, or intrathecal chemotherapy, which is injected directly into the cerebrospinal fluid. Intrathecal chemotherapy is commonly used to reduce the risk of cancer cells spreading to the central nervous system. If the cancer cells have spread to the central nervous system or are only in one specific area of the body, such as the testicles, then radiation therapy is also used in combination with chemotherapy. In addition to chemotherapy and radiation, antimetabolites, such as methotrexate and leucovorin, are often administered, as well as vincristine and prednisone at certain phases of treatment. Bone marrow or stem cell transplants are used for children whose prognosis of successful treatment is poor with chemotherapy and radiation (American Cancer Society, 2009).

Given the significant advances in the treatment of leukemia that have occurred over the past few decades and the considerable increase in survival rate, much attention is now focusing on the late effects of leukemia treatments. In particular, researchers have examined the long-term neuropsychological consequences of the intense treatments these children receive (Brown & Madan-Swain, 1993; Roman & Sperduto, 1995). The neurotoxicity associated with these treatments produces numerous permanent negative consequences, including central nervous system damage, leukoencephalopathy, neuroendocrine dysfunction, intracranial calcifications, demyelization, and cerebral atrophy (Picard & Rourke, 1995). White matter of the brain, which consists of myelinated neurons that conduct rapid transmission of brain signals required for cognitive functions, is significantly reduced in leukemia survivors, particularly in the right frontal regions (Carey et al., 2008). The damage resulting from these treatment methods has been found to affect learning, visuomotor ability, attention and memory, and intellectual ability.

Learning Outcomes

Van Dongen-Melman, De Groot, Van Dongen, Verhulst, and Hahlen (1997) investigated the effect of different types of central nervous system (CNS) prophylaxis on the leukemia survivors' identification by their school as having learning problems. They found that the 44% of the children who had been treated with CNS prophylaxis had significantly more learning problems than children who had not received CNS prophylaxis. Furthermore, they found that 80% of those who had received cranial irradiation with the CNS prophylaxis were identified by their school system as having learning problems.

Anderson, Smibert, Ekert, and Godber (1994) examined 100 leukemia survivors who had received chemotherapy in combination with radiation therapy, 50 survivors who had received chemotherapy without radiation, and 100 healthy control children chosen from Australian schools. Significant differences were revealed between the children who had received both chemotherapy and radiation and those who had received only chemotherapy or who were the healthy controls. Children treated with chemotherapy and radiation demonstrated the poorest educational skills of all three groups. This group achieved the lowest scores for reading, spelling, and arithmetic. The chemotherapy without radiation group and the control group, however, performed similarly on the educational achievement measures. This suggests that chemotherapy coupled with radiation results in the greatest late effects for academic achievement.

Waber and colleagues (1990) evaluated leukemia survivors who had received treatment including chemotherapy, cranial irradiation, and intrathecal methotrexate. They found that the leukemia survivors who had received cranial irradiation in their therapy achieved significantly poorer scores on reading and spelling tasks. In addition, females performed more poorly than males on an arithmetic and passage comprehension tasks. These findings suggest that treatment including irradiation appears to have a negative effect on later academic achievement skills. Radiation therapy may have a more pronounced negative impact on females' academic skills than on males'.

Attention and Memory

Another late effect of leukemia treatment on cognitive function appears to involve attention. Leukemia survivors demonstrate poorer performance on measures assessing the focus element of attention (Rodgers, Horrocks, Britton, & Kernahan, 1999). Children treated with cranial irradiation show significantly greater susceptibility to distraction and verbal memory (and the verbal memory deficits could be due to the problems of attention; Butler, Hill, Steinherz, Meyers, & Finlay, 1994). Brain scans of children receiving CNS prophylaxis reveal cortical atrophy and/or intracerebral calcifications caused by chemotherapy and cranial irradiation. Not surprisingly, children with abnormal brain scans exhibit poorer memory than those with normal scans (Brouwers & Poplack, 1990).

The attentional problems manifested by children receiving CNS prophylaxis may underlie their memory difficulties as well as the learning problems. The brain damage that results from treatment perpetuates the learning and attentional problems. Radiation therapy is believed to be the primary cause of the observed problems.

Cognitive Abilities

Researchers have examined the cognitive outcomes associated with leukemia treatment. Mulhern, Fairclough, and Ochs (1991) examined Full Scale IQs for childhood leukemia survivors and found only minimal and statistically nonsignificant changes in IQ. Other researchers have found that children who received chemotherapy and/or cranial irradiation obtained lower IQ scores than they did prior to radiation therapy (Silber et al., 1992). They also found that age at the time of irradiation seemed to affect IQ decline, in that the older the child was at the time of irradiation, the less the decline in IQ, with those under the age of 4 demonstrating the greatest decline.

Other researchers reported similar declines in intellectual ability for children treated with cranial irradiation (Jankovic & Brouwers, 1994; Schlieper, Esseltine, & Tarshis, 1989). However, when radiation treatment is not used, cognitive effects may be reduced. Children treated with only chemotherapy via intravenous methotrexate show no differences as compared to controls in their *accuracy* of information processing; however, they are *slower* on certain sustained attention and information-processing tasks (Mennes et al., 2005).

Gender Effects

In addition, significant sex differences have been found in children who receive radiation therapy, with girls performing significantly worse than boys for overall intellectual ability as well as performance ability (Schlieper et al., 1989). Girls with acute lymphoblastic leukemia receiving combined cranial radiation and chemotherapy or chemotherapy alone demonstrate verbal learning and auditory-verbal attention deficits when compared to healthy controls (Précourt et al., 2002). Similarly, intellectual declines have been found only for girls who were treated with chemotherapy and high-dose methotrexate in combination with cranial irradiation (Waber et al., 1995).

Research into visuomotor control deficits following chemotherapy confirms the gender effects associated with high-dose methotrexate treatment. Children with acute lymphoblastic leukemia treated with chemotherapy (without irradiation) evidence visuomotor deficits, and females and those with more recent chemotherapy treatment are particularly susceptible. Girls appear to be at a particularly high risk for visuomotor deficits resulting from high-dose methotrexate treatment (Buizer, De Sonneville, Van Den Heuvel-Eibrink, Njiokikjien, & Veerman, 2005).

Overall, the research indicates that there may be late effects of intellectual decline; however, it is not entirely clear as to whether the decline occurs mainly in the area of performance-related tasks or more globally. Research also suggests that age at treatment, as well as the gender of the child, may be important factors that influence the degree of impact. The amount of methotrexate used in treatment may play a role in addition whether cranial irradiation is used. For example, difficulties in working memory and nonverbal skills emerge during the first year of intravenous methotrexate treatment, and severity of difficulties relates to methotrexate dosage and/or infusion rate (Carey et al., 2007).

IMPLICATIONS FOR EDUCATORS

The considerable increase in survival rates of childhood leukemia over the past several decades makes it more likely that school professionals will work with these children during their career. Surviving children commonly enter or re-enter the school system following treatment and remission of the disease (Brown & Madan-Swain, 1993). Rather than requiring an extended hospital stay, many children are receiving treatments on an outpatient basis and attending school at the same time. Therefore, knowledge of the effects of leukemia treatments is important for educators. Educators should be alert to potential problems related to learning, attention, memory, and intellectual ability that may surface following treatment. Awareness of the child's medical status and active daily monitoring allow for early identification of learning problems and subsequent intervention. The educational team may want to request medical information regarding the child's treatment to assess whether irradiation and methotrexate treatment was used, which may portend more severe neuropsychological effects. The team should consider the age and gender of the child as well, as younger children and girls are more likely to have long-term effects.

Up to 40% of children with leukemia may have reoccurrence of the disease (Lampkin, DeLaat, & George, 1992), which means that the school also needs to prepare for the possibility of numerous school absences and the need for alternate instruction. Although school attendance is desired, even for half-days, educators should be prepared to organize instructional efforts and facilitate communication among family at home, school staff, and medical personnel should home- or hospital-based instruction be required. School psychologists may need to conduct psychoeducational assessments to ascertain whether the child qualifies for additional supportive services under the Other Health Impaired classification. If difficulties persist beyond the expertise of the school psychologist and other school personnel, then a referral to a neuropsychologist familiar with the neuropsychological effects of leukemia and its treatments is recommended.

Emotional and coping supports are important for the long-term success of surviving children. Childhood cancer survivors may benefit from counseling services, which address both their transition back into the school setting and the stress they experience as a result of their disease and treatment (Robaey et al., 2000). Educators should be particularly sensitive to the child's parents, who may be extremely anxious after facing this life-threatening illness with their child, signing consent forms for treatments that threaten to inflict long-term damage due to side effects, and suffering through their child's long, often painful treatment (Zins, Ponti, & Noll, 1998). Educators are called upon to exercise compassion, empathy, and common sense when communicating with parents, particularly with regard to academic rules, regulations, and expectations.

Education about leukemia for fellow students and other teachers in the school may prove useful in reducing the stigma the students feel because of a lack of information or misinformation regarding childhood cancer. It is important for the child's peers and teachers to convey a sense of optimism regarding his or her recovery and long-term potential. In addition, teachers may need to understand the physiological effects resulting from ongoing or recently completed treatment, such as hair loss, weight fluctuation, fatigue, cognitive impairments, motor difficulties, and possible social and emotional complications like the fear of death (Zins et al., 1998). The child's ability to recovery socially and re-engage with his or her peer group following a sustained absence and physiological changes is paramount, and school personnel should be ready to accommodate the student in this regard (e.g., by allowing the child to wear a hat or providing more frequent breaks).

Educational strategies such as teaching students to use their cognitive strengths to compensate for attentional and memory deficits may prove helpful (Anderson et al., 1994). Armstrong et al. (1999) suggested using tools such as books-on-tape and computer-based voice recognition software to ameliorate problems related to visual memory, visual-motor integration, processing speed, and fine-motor speed. Untimed testing, oral assessment, and calculator use for mathematics may also be beneficial accommodations. The use of psychostimulants (e.g., methylphenidate) can be helpful in improving attention, cognitive flexibility, and processing speed (Conklin et al., 2007). It is important to remember, however, that interventions must be made on a case-by-case basis, because each child may have varying levels of impairment following treatment and survival. The best intervention is prevention of academic and social difficulties, so assessing and addressing potential problems is the best practice when working with childhood cancer survivors.

EDUCATIONAL STRATEGIES

- More children are surviving childhood leukemia, and they may be receiving treatment on an outpatient basis rather than during an extended hospital stay. This means that the child may be attending school while receiving treatment. Educators are encouraged to stay in close contact with the family and medical team so as to be prepared for treatment effects.
- Measurement of baseline functioning is important as a means to assess the effects of leukemia treatments. Educators can conduct a thorough evaluation of academic skills prior to admission for treatment. School psychologists can conduct a full psychological battery, including cognitive, visuomotor, attention, and memory tests. With this information, it is then possible to assess whether the child has any late effects caused by treatments. This information should be shared with the medical team and family.
- Given that around 40% of children with leukemia have recurrence, it is important that the educational team plan ahead to anticipate school absences and alternate instruction.
- It is important to educate the child's classmates about leukemia and the treatment procedure so they understand what is happening and can be supportive of the child. Providing such information also helps to reduce stigma and mistruths associated with disease (e.g., it is not contagious) and helps to convey optimism about recovery.
- Emotional and coping supports are important for the long-term success of surviving children and their families. Treatments and side effects can be painful and stressful. Educators are encouraged to exercise compassion, empathy, and common sense when communicating with parents, particularly with regard to academic rules and regulations.
- Teaching students to use their cognitive strengths to compensate for attention and memory deficits is helpful. Problems related to visual memory, visual-motor integration, processing speed, and fine-motor speed are possible following treatment. Untimed testing, oral assessment, books-on-tape, voice recognition software, and calculator use may be useful accommodations.

DISCUSSION QUESTIONS

1. What, if anything, should be shared with the ill child and his or her class about the diagnosis of leukemia and possibility of death?

2. What might be the child's age-appropriate concerns about the disease and treatment?

3. What steps can schools take to assist families with a child with leukemia?

4. Since medical treatments are increasingly conducted on an outpatient basis, what should schools do to prepare for the re-entry of a child with a chronic illness like leukemia?

5. Cognitive effects of treatments can be mistaken for laziness, oppositional behavior, or noncompliance. How can educators distinguish neuropsychological effects from other behavioral problems?

RESEARCH SUMMARY

- Leukemia is a cancer of white blood cells that originates in the bone marrow and can then spread to the blood, lymph nodes, central nervous system, and organs.
- Children identified as having leukemia usually have either acute lymphocytic leukemia or acute myelogenous leukemia. Acute lymphocytic leukemia, a cancer of the lymphocyte-forming cells, is the most common type of childhood leukemia. Acute myelogenous leukemia is a cancer of the bone marrow cells that form granulocytes, monocytes, red blood cells, and platelets.
- Leukemia accounts for approximately one third of all cancers in children under the age of 15 and approximately one fourth of all cancers in those less than 20 years of age.
- Acute lymphocyte leukemia is most often diagnosed in early childhood, peaking between 2 and 4 years of age, while acute myelogenous is diagnosed throughout childhood with slight peaks before age 2 and during adolescence. Over 91% of children under 5 survive acute lymphocytic leukemia, and just over 60% of children under age 15 survive acute myelogenous leukemia.
- The treatment for childhood leukemia usually consists of 2 to 3 years of intense drug therapy. Children with leukemia typically receive either systemic chemotherapy, which is usually administered intravenously, or intrathecal chemotherapy, which is injected directly into the cerebrospinal fluid. If the cancer cells have spread to the central nervous system or are in one specific area of the body, then radiation therapy is also used in combination with chemotherapy. Bone marrow or stem cell transplants are used for children who do not respond to chemotherapy and radiation.
- The neurotoxicity resulting from these treatments can produce permanent damage to the central nervous system, leading to negative consequences associated with learning, visuomotor ability, attention and memory, and intellectual ability.
- Younger children and girls appear to be at particular risk for greater long-term negative effects of treatment, especially from irradiation. The amount of methotrexate used in treatment may play a role in addition to the use of cranial irradiation.

RESOURCES

American Cancer Society: www.cancer.org

Kidshealth.org (For Parents): http://kidshealth.org/parent/medical/cancer/cancer_leukemia.html

The Leukemia & Lymphoma Society: www.leukemia-lymphoma.org

HANDOUT

COGNITIVE EFFECTS OF LEUKEMIA TREATMENTS

Cancer is the term used to describe a category of diseases in which cells in the body mutate and multiply. Although the occurrence of cancer in children and adolescents is relatively rare in comparison to its occurrence in adults, cancer is the second leading cause of death in children age 14 and under.

Leukemia is a cancer of the white blood cells. This form of cancer originates in the bone marrow and can then spread to the blood, lymph nodes, central nervous system, and organs. Children identified as having leukemia have either acute lymphocytic leukemia or acute myelogenous leukemia. Acute lymphocytic leukemia, a cancer of the lymphocyte-forming cells (which are B-cells or T-cells), is the most common type of childhood leukemia. Acute myelogenous leukemia is a cancer of the bone marrow cells that form granulocytes, monocytes, red blood cells, and platelets.

More than 95% of children with acute lymphocytic leukemia now enter remission after one month of treatment. It is also estimated that the long-term survival rate for children with leukemia is currently greater than 70%. Over 91% of children under 5 survive acute lymphocytic leukemia, and just over 60% of children under age 15 survive acute myelogenous leukemia. Given these higher survival rates, researchers are now focusing on the long-term neuropsychological consequences of the powerful treatments used to eradicate the cancer.

Treatments for Leukemia

- The treatment for childhood leukemia usually consists of 2 to 3 years of intense drug therapy. Children with leukemia typically receive either systemic chemotherapy, which is usually administered intravenously, or intrathecal chemotherapy, which is injected directly into the cerebrospinal fluid.
- If the cancer cells have spread to the central nervous system or are only in one specific area of the body, radiation therapy is used in combination with chemotherapy.
- In addition to chemotherapy and radiation, antimetabolites such as methotrexate and leucovorin are often given, as well as vincristine and prednisone at certain phases of treatment.
- Bone marrow or stem cell transplants are used for children whose prognosis of successful treatment is poor with chemotherapy.

Cognitive Effects

- The neurotoxicity associated with these treatments produces numerous permanent negative consequences, which may include the following:
  - Central nervous system damage
  - Leukoencephalopathy
  - Neuroendocrine dysfunction
  - Intracranial calcifications
  - Cerebral atrophy
- The damage to the central nervous system resulting from these treatment methods has been found to impact the following:
  - Learning
  - Visuomotor ability
  - Attention and memory
  - Intellectual ability, especially evident in a slowing of information processing

It is important for parents and teachers to work together to assist the child during and after leukemia treatments to mitigate their negative side effects. Accommodations may need to be made at home and at school to help the child meet expectations for behavior and learning. In addition, several simple steps can help the child readjust successfully:

- School personnel should be educated on the illness and alerted to the potential problems related to learning, attention, memory, and intellectual ability that may surface.
- The educational team can assess the child to obtain baseline levels of functioning so the long-term effects of treatment can be measured.
- The age and gender of the child are important, because younger children and girls are more likely to evidence long-term negative effects from treatment (especially irradiation).
- Up to 40% of children with leukemia may have recurrence of the disease, which means that the school needs to prepare for the possibility of numerous school absences and the need for alternate instruction.
- Childhood cancer survivors may benefit from counseling services to address their transition back into the school setting, as well as to relieve the stress they experience because of their disease and treatment.
- Education about leukemia for fellow students and other teachers in the school may prove useful in reducing stigma; conveying a sense of optimism regarding the child's recovery and long-term potential; and explaining physiological effects resulting from ongoing or recently completed treatment, such as hair loss, weight fluctuation, fatigue, cognitive impairments, motor difficulties, and possible social and emotional complications like the fear of death.

8

An Overview of Pediatric Human Immunodeficiency Virus (HIV)*

Sarah A. Bassin, W. Mark Posey, and Emily E. Powell

A 5-year-old boy, Tyrone, has just been referred to the Intervention Assistance Team, with the psychologist as the case manager. The child demonstrates borderline cognitive ability and delayed fine motor skills. In addition, he experiences speech/language difficulties as well as symptoms of attention deficit/hyperactivity disorder (ADHD). The child's achievement is delayed. He has been hospitalized once for pneumonia; has had other, recurrent health problems, including sore throats and ear infections; and is small for his age. Tyrone's life has been chaotic, with his father incarcerated and his mother moving more than once a year due to difficulties in paying rent. Recently, he moved in with his grandmother so that he does not change schools each time his mother moves.

This description reveals a number of risk factors that are likely contributing to Tyrone's difficulties. However, in reviewing the case with the grandparent, the school psychologist suggested that there might be a medical explanation for the child's difficulties, including a genetic or other health condition that could have been passed on to him by his parents, and recommended that they consult with the child's pediatrician. The pediatrician conducted a number of blood tests, including an HIV test, and the child tested positive for HIV. Initially, the child's grandmother and mother did not believe the diagnosis. The pediatrician referred the family to a pediatrician who specializes in infectious diseases, and a social worker in the office assisted the family in working through their anger and grief.

*Adapted from Wilson, S., & Posey, M. (2007). Pediatric Human Immunodeficiency Virus (HIV): Overview and developmental effects. *Communiqué, 36*(4), 27–29. Copyright by the National Association of School Psychologists, Bethesda, MD. Use is by permission of the publisher. www.nasponline.org

After several months of being in a stable, loving home environment with his grandmother, attending appointments with the pediatric infectious disease specialist and his staff, and adhering to the medication regimen, Tyrone's behavior and learning at school began to improve. In addition, he began speech therapy at school. Tyrone's grandmother has not disclosed his status to the school psychologist yet, but they remain in contact regarding his progress.

INTRODUCTION

HIV stands for human immunodeficiency virus: a virus that targets the immune system. The virus specifically attacks and destroys CD4 cells. These are white blood cells that are important for effective immune system functioning. As a child's CD4 count decreases, immune system functioning declines. Consequently, the child becomes more susceptible to potentially life-threatening infections and ultimately develops acquired immunodeficiency syndrome (AIDS). Students with HIV are at risk for a wide range of cognitive, language, neurological, and social-emotional difficulties with corresponding needs for special services in school.

Children infected with HIV usually contract the virus due to vertical infection from the mother, either prenatally, perinatally, or postnatally. Perinatal infection, often related to breast-feeding, accounts for more than 84% of cases in children less than 13 years old at diagnosis (CDC, 2007). Once children are infected, the disease progresses through four categories (American Academy of Pediatrics, 2003). The first is Category N, which includes children who only exhibit one symptom of mild HIV or no symptoms. The second stage is called Category A, which includes children who are mildly symptomatic. Symptoms may include swelling of glands and organs or chronic inflammation and infection of the upper respiratory system, sinuses, and middle ear. The third stage is called Category B, which includes children who are moderately symptomatic. A large number of symptoms may characterize this stage, including persistent low levels of hemoglobin; a single episode of a severe infection, such as bacterial meningitis or pneumonia; or chronic herpes outbreaks. The fourth and final stage of symptoms is called Category C, which includes children who are severely symptomatic. Symptoms may include wasting syndrome; progressive encephalopathy; cancers; and serious infections, such as tuberculosis (American Academy of Pediatrics).

BACKGROUND

Scope of the Problem

Of children infected with HIV, 90% will experience developmental delays without medical intervention (Renwick, Goldie, & King, 2007). Even with appropriate care, most of these children eventually experience cognitive and motoric developmental delays or regression (American Academy of Pediatrics, 2003; Wachsler-Felder & Golden, 2002).

Because of children's immature nervous systems, pediatric HIV can cause extensive neuropsychological and developmental deficits beyond those effects experienced by adults (Wachsler-Felder & Golden, 2002). The level of cognitive impairment correlates with the stage of HIV disease, which is affected by treatment quality and medication adherence (Brouwers, Wolters, & Civitello, 1998). Appropriate treatment, increased CD4 cell count, and reduced viral load are associated with fewer deficits in functioning (Jeremy et al., 2005; Wachsler-Felder & Golden).

Although the most serious neuropsychological symptoms are associated with the final stage of HIV, developmental delays are often detected prior to this stage. Neuropsychological effects vary from children who function within normal limits to children with encephalopathy (Brouwers, Wolters, & Civitello, 1998). For example, a recent report of functioning in 298 clinically stable HIV-infected children ranging in age from 2 to 17 years old found frequent behavioral problems as well as lower developmental and cognitive scores compared to those of their age peers (Nozyce et al., 2006). Broad areas of development that may be affected by these brain abnormalities include motor development, general cognitive functioning, language skills, and executive functioning.

Motor Development and Visual–Motor Effects of HIV

According to Englund and colleagues (1996), neuropsychological abnormalities in children with HIV commonly involve motor deficits. More recently, using the Bayley Scales of Infant Development II (Bayley II), Nozyce and colleagues (2006) found that the mean Motor Development Index for infants and toddlers with HIV was 78, whereas the average score for the general population is 100. In addition, Jeremy and colleagues (2005) found that viral load is associated with performance on fine motor tasks involving both hands but not single-hand tasks. Others have also found a significant difference between infected and uninfected young children in their motor development, whether or not their treatment regimen included highly active antiretroviral therapy (HAART; Lindsey, Malee, Brouwers, & Hughes, 2007). However, results from the Bayley II suggest mild improvements in children's motor skills after beginning HAART (Lindsey et al.). HAART usually involves a combination of several different medications that interferes with HIV's ability to copy itself and reduces HIV's concentration in the blood. This decrease in HIV concentration is important, because lower viral load is associated with a lower risk of disease progression, including neuropsychological effects.

In the final stage of the disease, when children begin to experience encephalopathy, they may also demonstrate gross motor symptoms, such as toe-walking, overactive reflexes, and augmented muscle tone in the legs, which may affect their gait (Wachsler-Felder & Golden, 2002). Consequently, children with HIV are likely to have trouble in school with tasks dependent on fine motor and visual-motor skills, such as using scissors or writing.

Cognitive Effects

Pediatric HIV also affects cognitive outcomes. Given these difficulties, it is not surprising that 40% of children with HIV receive special education services (Rutstein et al., 2007). Cognitive ability is associated with viral load and CD4 count (Jeremy et al., 2005; Shanbhag et al., 2005). In fact, the likelihood of cognitive delay appears specifically related to viral load in the months immediately after birth (Wachsler-Felder & Golden, 2002). This finding supports the importance of early medical intervention.

Even children with a very low viral load continue to demonstrate decreased neuropsychological performance compared to standardization samples (Jeremy et al., 2005). Similar to results from the Motor Development Index, scores from the Mental Development Index of the Bayley II are lower for infants and toddlers with HIV, with one study finding a mean cognitive standard score of 76 and another reporting a mean standard score of 65 (Nozyce et al., 2006). Again, the average score on these assessments is 100.

Other research suggests cognitive benefits related to the initiation of HAART. One study comparing children's cognitive scores pre- and post-HAART found an average increase of 4.9 in cognitive ability after the use of HAART ($M = 100$, $SD = 15$; Shanbhag et al., 2005). The implementation of HAART was also associated with a decrease in progressive and static encephalopathy, both of which are associated with a significant decrease in measured cognitive ability. Another study found that children's average decline in cognitive ability after HAART slowed from 8.4 points per year to 1.1 points per year, as measured on the Bayley II (Lindsey et al., 2007). Thus, while children with HIV are likely to experience cognitive deficits that can affect their ability to learn at the same rate as their peers, there is some evidence that HAART mitigates these effects.

Language Development

Language functioning may also be affected in children with HIV (e.g., Blanchette, Smith, King, Fernandes-Penney, & Read, 2002). One study reported that children with HIV experience deficits in receptive and expressive language that increase with time; however, receptive language is better developed than expressive language (Wachsler-Felder & Golden, 2002). Although the results suggest that these effects are unrelated to antiretroviral treatment, much of this research occurred prior to the implementation of HAART, which may decrease these language deficits through its apparent positive effect on cognitive outcomes (Shanbhag et al., 2005). Still, children with HIV are at risk for language delays, particularly in expressive language, which can negatively influence the development of their social skills and can affect other behaviors that impact learning, such as their willingness to speak in the classroom.

Executive Functioning

There is evidence for the effects of HIV on attention and executive functioning, as well as on general cognitive ability and language. For example, as of 1997, children with HIV demonstrated more behaviors associated with attention deficit/hyperactivity disorder (ADHD) than uninfected children ("Antiretroviral," 1998; "1997 USPHS/IDSA," 1998). In fact, the prevalence of ADHD in children with HIV has been estimated at 20%, a rate higher than that associated with chronic health conditions in general (Nozyce et al., 2006). Furthermore, in 2000, Watkins and colleagues (2000) found that the performance of children with HIV on a task involving concentration decreased relative to their uninfected peers the longer they had to concentrate. However, this effect became less pronounced in older children (Wachsler-Felder & Golden, 2002). In addition, Bisiacchi, Suppeij, and Laverda (2000) found executive functioning difficulties in all of the infected children they assessed, across all stages of infection. Therefore, children with HIV are likely to experience attention and executive difficulties that can affect their ability to access the curriculum. In addition, these difficulties may also be interpreted as behavior problems in the classroom.

Psychosocial Adjustment

Psychological well-being is an important aspect of all children's development. Adequate psychological adjustment is particularly critical for children with HIV, given the evidence of a connection between physical health and depressive symptoms in individuals with HIV (Yi et al., 2006). In addition, a recent review found that psychological interventions were positively related to immune system functioning across a variety of pediatric chronic health conditions, including HIV (Nassau, Tien, & Fritz, 2008). For any child with a chronic health problem, psychological risk factors are determined not only by the course of the condition but also by child, family, and environmental factors. However, HIV is somewhat different from other pediatric chronic health conditions in that disease effects are frequently intimately intertwined with many psychosocial risk factors. Some risk factors in addition to the disease itself are poor nutrition, poor health/death of a primary caregiver, familial instability, low SES, maternal education, single parenting, parental drug use or other risk behaviors, prenatal drug exposure, or ethnic group status. Fathers may be absent, incarcerated, or uninvolved (Smith, Martin, & Wolters, 2004). Many of these negative environmental factors are risk factors for delays in cognitive development, as well as for psychological well-being.

Risk factors more directly due to the health condition include the social stigma associated with HIV, as well as an uncertain future involving ongoing adherence to complex medications and an increasingly limited ability to participate in enjoyable activities (Roberts, 2000). In teenagers, issues of sexual development are compounded by the child having a sexually transmitted infection (Smith et al., 2004). Consequently, psychologists and school staff must consider the availability of a support system for the child and the family and the effects of loss, stress, grief, and anger on the child and family members.

Some research also suggests that children with HIV are at risk for psychological adjustment problems. The literature indicates concerns with anxiety and depression and behaviors ranging from apathy and withdrawal to suicidal ideation (Roberts, 2000). In our clinical experience, possible passive suicide has been observed, involving refusal to comply with medication regimens. One multisite study with 839 participants found that

13.3% of children with HIV demonstrated emotional, social, and/or behavioral difficulties (Englund et al., 1996). Depressive disorders are also more common among adolescents with HIV, and 82% of adolescents with HIV in one study struggled with substance abuse and half were a victim of sexual abuse (Pao et al., 2000).

Disclosure

One of the most important social-emotional issues all children with HIV must address is disclosure. State laws and school district policies regarding HIV disclosure vary. In one sample of 92 school-aged children, 53% had not disclosed their status to the school. For those children who had disclosed their status, school nurses were most frequently told, followed by principals and then teachers (Cohen et al., 1997).

Parents must decide not only when to disclose to the child but also when to disclose within the community. Many parents are hesitant to disclose an HIV diagnosis to the child because HIV is associated with many stigmatized behaviors, such as drug use. Many parents are afraid that their child will resent and reject them for passing on the virus and for engaging in risky behaviors. Many parents plan to tell their child at some point but wait because they do not want to harm their child, they want their child to remain innocent, or they do not think that their child is old enough to understand (Gerson et al., 2001).

There are three types of disclosure: nondisclosure, partial disclosure, and full disclosure. In nondisclosure, children are not told that they have an illness. Instead, parents may explain the pill regime as "vitamins" or necessary for a "lung condition." In partial disclosure, children are told that they have an illness but are not told that they have HIV, and they are not told all of the information about their illness. They often are informed that they need to take their medicine to control their illness and that they have a "germ" in their blood so they should not let anyone touch it. Finally, in full disclosure, children are told that they have HIV and are told specific details about their condition. There is little agreement in the literature concerning the percentage of children who have partial disclosure or full disclosure; however, trends suggest that older children, children with higher IQs, and children with lower CD4 counts are more likely to have full disclosure (Mellins, Richards, Nicholas, & Abrams, 2002; Wiener, Mellins, Marhefka, & Battles, 2007).

Despite parents' concerns about the potential detrimental effects of partial or full disclosure, most of the literature indicates various positive outcomes. In fact, the American Academy of Pediatrics (1999) recommends disclosure, although not a specific age at which to disclose. Research suggests that disclosure does not result in increased mental health problems and may even lessen depressive symptoms (Mellins et al., 2001). Additionally, children who have experienced full disclosure are more likely to have higher self-esteem and have a better understanding of their medical condition than those experiencing no or partial disclosure (Bose, Moss, Brouwers, Pizzo, & Lorion, 1994; Funck-Brentano et al., 1997). In contrast, nondisclosure is associated with psychological maladjustment, as well as caregiver and family stress (Bachanas et al., 2001).

IMPLICATIONS FOR EDUCATORS

If we use the same universal precautions with all children, then there is no need for children with HIV to be treated any differently than other children in the school setting. More and more children with HIV will enter our schools, as life expectancy and quality of life improve with the development of increasingly effective HAART medications. As the number of affected children who attend schools grows, the likelihood that we will serve them will also increase, and we will have opportunities for interactions that may help mitigate the stigma associated with HIV infection. Given the positive effects of prevention and intervention on development, all of us must work together to overcome this perceived stigma and communicate a message of hope to these children and their families.

EDUCATIONAL STRATEGIES

- Monitor students' physical symptoms and invite physicians' involvement when appropriate.
- Consider the child's family and social support network in terms of how they can help promote adherence to the treatment regimen.
- Consider child and family grief and how these emotions might impact the child's behavior and learning at home and at school.
- Plan for intermittent absences from school.
- HIV can affect a child's brain development, resulting in a range of negative effects. Expect and plan for differentiation in terms of instruction and behavioral management due to difficulties with gross and fine motor skills, limitations in reasoning abilities, difficulties understanding and using language, and behavioral problems that overlap with ADHD.

DISCUSSION QUESTIONS

1. What are some difficulties for parents whose children have HIV?

2. Because of these difficulties, why are support systems so important for these families?

3. What are some issues to consider with the three levels of disclosure listed in this chapter?

4. How would you talk to a parent about helping a child maintain the medication regimen?

5. How would you discuss the disease with the child affected by HIV at age 6 versus age 12 versus age 17?

RESEARCH SUMMARY

- Children's level of general cognitive impairment is correlated with the stage of HIV disease, which is affected by treatment quality and medication adherence.

- Children with HIV may be at increased risk for difficulties with psychological adjustment.
- Effective treatment, decreased viral load, and increased CD4 cell count have correlated with more positive developmental outcomes.
- Children with HIV are more likely to drop out of school and more likely to be unemployed compared to national norms (Battles & Wiener, 2002).
- Children who receive full disclosure generally demonstrate better adjustment.
- Social support may also serve as a protective factor, as increased social support is related to decreased behavior problems (Battles & Wiener, 2002).
- Protective factors in general may be related to having adequate access to social-emotional and medical resources.

RESOURCES

Brochures from the Centers for Disease Control and Prevention: www.cdc.gov/hiv/resources/brochures/index.htm

Community resources for children with HIV: www.vachss.com/help_text/hiv_aids_ped.html#org

HANDOUT

PEDIATRIC HIV

What Is HIV?

- Human immunodeficiency virus is a virus that targets the immune system and leads to developmental problems for children.
- HIV is a progressive disease, but it is now viewed as a chronic health condition due to significant improvements in treatment.

Potential Negative Effects on Thinking Abilities and Related Skills

- Fine motor difficulties (small muscles)
- Gross motor symptoms (large muscles) in later stages of the illness
- Below-average scores for cognitive development (or thinking abilities)
- Difficulties understanding and using language
- Problems involving hyperactivity, impulsivity, and inattention
- Effects are related to the amount of virus and number of white blood cells (CD4) in the blood.
- Better adherence to treatment regimens helps limit developmental effects.

Psychosocial Effects

- Parents and caregivers are dealing with difficult issues, and this may impact the child.
  - Isolation may occur due to the social stigma of HIV.
  - Limited financial and social resources may decrease options for social support.
  - Research strongly suggests that parents whose children have HIV have decreased options for social support than other parents.
- Given results suggesting decreased social support for these families, involvement of the school, other family members, and mental health professionals is very important.
- The school needs to keep in mind that children must often adjust to transitions between homes due to parental difficulties.
- Children may have trouble with anxiety and/or depression related to their condition. These difficulties may be worsened if other family members have mental health issues as well.
- Disclosure can support improved adjustment for children, but this is a very personal family decision.
  - Enlist the help of other professionals (school psychologist, family physician, social worker, and/or other physicians) who are intimately involved with the child's care.

Additional Risk Factors

Consider factors related to low socioeconomic status, often associated with HIV, that may negatively affect development, such as nutrition, the stress of inconsistent employment or insufficient income, or a changing home environment.

9

Bacterial Meningitis*

Paul C. McCabe and Fallon Lattari

Keisha was a first-grade student with a charming and sociable personality. She was popular with students in her grade and eager to please her teacher. Keisha did well in school, achieving average grades and demonstrating mastery of basic reading and math concepts. She was only occasionally distractible and no more so than her classmates. Shortly before concluding her first-grade year, Keisha became sick with a fever of over 102 degrees. Her parents tended to her symptoms with a pain reliever on the advice of a pediatrician. Keisha's fever lowered slightly, but she quickly became lethargic and despondent. After 2 days, Keisha was taken to the hospital.

Keisha immediately underwent a battery of tests to determine her medical and mental status. She appeared comatose, failing to respond to any sensory stimuli. Her functioning indicated symptoms of neurological impairment. Keisha had contracted bacterial meningitis and encephalitis, and she spent 2 weeks in the intensive care unit and another 2 weeks in rehabilitation. A neuropsychological evaluation was completed toward the end of her hospital stay to assess any residual deficits. Keisha presented with attention difficulties, response inhibition difficulties, executive functioning deficits, and visual and perceptual problems that impacted on reading, writing, and spelling skills. Her performance led to diagnoses of developmental coordination disorder, attention deficit/hyperactivity disorder (inattentive type), and developmental reading disorder.

Keisha slowly transitioned back to school following rehabilitation, gradually increasing the length of her school day. It was noted that she was disorganized, highly distracted, and engaged in atypical behaviors, which included licking and chewing. She was often not able to apply what she had learned, and she sought

(Continued)

*Adapted from Kelly, H., & McCabe, P. C. (2004). Bacterial meningitis: What school psychologists need to know. *Communiqué, 32*(5), 37–39. Copyright by the National Association of School Psychologists, Bethesda, MD. Use is by permission of the publisher. www.nasponline.org

(Continued)

the attention of adults. Academically, Keisha struggled with skills that she had previously mastered. She demonstrated tracking problems; sensory processing deficits; information processing difficulties; decreased fine motor, visual motor, and handwriting skills; and inconsistency in blending sounds when reading. She also worked at an extremely slow pace, frequently took mental breaks by getting out of her seat, and regularly sought sensory input. She was referred to the Committee on Special Education, and it was recommended that she participate in a remedial class for language arts and math and receive occupational therapy and consultant teacher support for mainstream academics.

INTRODUCTION

Meningitis is a condition in which the meninges, which are protective membranes surrounding the brain and spinal cord, become infected and inflamed, possibly leading to neurological damage. Meningitis can be caused by a bacterial, viral, fungal, or parasitic infection. Viral meningitis is diagnosed almost exclusively in children under age 5, while bacterial meningitis is more typically diagnosed among preteens, adolescents, and adults due to the success of recent vaccinations of young children (CDC, 2009). Bacterial meningitis, the most noxious of the varieties, is associated with comparatively high rates of morbidity and mortality despite advances in medical care. Before the use of antibiotic treatments for bacterial meningitis, the fatality rate was nearly 100% (Michael, 2002). Current estimates are that 10% to 15% of all cases are fatal and that 10% to 15% of survivors have long-term neurological damage, such as permanent hearing loss (CDC). Over 25% of survivors have significant neuropsychological effects, including sensorineural, learning, and behavioral problems, and many of these difficulties are not evident until a child is school-aged (Grimwood et al., 1995). Educators play an important role in the management and support of children who have suffered from meningitis, both immediately after discharge as well as throughout the school years.

BACKGROUND

Pathogenesis

The forms of meningococci bacteria that cause meningitis are commonly found in the mucous that lines the nose, throat, and tonsils. Disease occurs only when this bacteria comes into contact with another strain of meningococci bacteria acquired either directly from an infected individual or indirectly from an infection in another part of the body, as occurs with some postoperative patients (Weir, 2002). Infants may acquire pathogens during birth by contact and aspiration of intestinal and genital tract secretions from the mother, although they do not exclusively become sick in this way. Newborns can also be exposed to multiple nosocomial pathogens during extended exposure to other newborns (Sáez-Llorens & McCracken, 2003). Many of the organisms that cause meningitis in infants and children colonize the upper respiratory tract.

Risk factors for meningitis include immunodeficiency disorders, such as AIDS; recent respiratory tract infections; exposure to cigarette smoke; and overcrowded living conditions. Other factors include penetrating head injuries, neurosurgical procedures, or cerebrospinal fluid (CSF) leaks. Populations most commonly affected by bacterial meningitis are infants and young children; elderly adults; and large groups that share facilities, such as dormitory students. There is also evidence that recipients of cochlear implants are at a 30-fold increased risk for contracting bacterial meningitis (Chavez-Bueno & McCracken, 2005). Additionally, researchers believe that illnesses or environmental conditions, such as dry air, could contribute to the thinning and damage of mucus membranes and increase susceptibility to the disease. Evidence for this hypothesis is the greater prevalence of bacterial meningitis during the late winter and early spring (Michael, 2002).

Once the pathogenic bacteria penetrate the mucus membrane layer, they can invade the blood-brain barrier, contaminate the bloodstream, and spread throughout the meninges and tissue that surrounds the brain. Within the meninges, the bacteria replicate rapidly, every 20 to 30 minutes, in the subarachnoid space and cause significant swelling and intracranial pressure. White blood cells also begin to accumulate in the CSF and contribute an inflammatory response (Phillips & Simor, 1998). In addition, the walls of the blood vessels themselves become inflamed, leading to decreased blood flow. The swelling of these tissues, referred to as *edema*, causes a temporary deficiency of blood flow. Because bacteria and white blood cells can obstruct the flow of CSF, proper drainage and circulation is hindered, which contributes to edema, and further constriction of blood flow. When the brain lacks blood and oxygen supply, neurons die (Michael, 2002).

Clinical Symptoms

Given the higher incidence rates of bacterial meningitis among infants and young children, who typically cannot verbalize their discomfort, it is crucial to recognize the symptoms of meningitis. However, manifestations of the condition depend on the age of the patient. The signs and symptoms of bacterial meningitis are generally more subtle and atypical among younger patients. In children, signs of meningitis may include fever, lethargy, behavioral changes, arching of the back, refusal of food, vomiting, a bulging fontanel ("soft spot" of the head), seizures, and, in about half of child cases, a deep red or purple rash ("Meningitis in Children," 1999; Parini, 2002). Seizures occur in about one third of children with bacterial meningitis.

A study examining the course of clinical features of meningococcal disease in children and adolescents before admission to a hospital identified three early signs of the illness, generally appearing within the first 12 hours (Thompson et al., 2006). These include leg pain, cold hands and feet, and abnormal skin color. Symptoms progress rapidly, over a period of a few hours, and can be followed by extreme drowsiness or lack of consciousness ("Meningitis in Children," 1999). Classic meningitis symptoms include fever, severe headache, stiffness of the neck, nausea or vomiting, sensitivity to light, and changes in mental status (Parini, 2002). Because these more classic symptoms usually occur later in the prehospital illness, parents are encouraged to examine their sick child for all possible signs of the disease and consult a doctor if the child's condition worsens.

Neurological Effects

The types and extent of brain injury caused by bacterial meningitis depend on the severity of individual cases, host factors such as immune functioning, and the timeliness of diagnosis and treatment. The most significant cause of neuronal injury is intracranial pressure, because it causes diffuse, widespread, and focal, localized cortical damage. As a result, a diverse cascade of neuropsychological outcomes is associated with bacterial meningitis. Frequently cited conditions include sensorineural hearing loss, hemiparesis (paralysis of one side of the body), seizure disorders, cranial nerve palsies, mild to moderate intellectual disabilities, motor deficits, moderate to severe developmental delay, learning difficulties, blindness, speech and language disabilities, and behavioral problems (Chinchankar et al., 2002). Research indicates that about 10% to 15% of the children who survive the disease suffer from such complications and up to 20% experience long-term cognitive, academic, and behavioral problems (Koomen et al., 2005). Bacterial meningitis has a particularly devastating effect on the developing central nervous system and the formation of neural connections.

Reduced neural complexity, found in infant rats afflicted with the disease, as well as hippocampal atrophy found in surviving humans, account for frequently observed learning deficits among infected individuals (Guerra-Romero, Tureen, & Tauber, 1992; Nau & Bruck, 2002). Infected infants were found to evidence significant learning disabilities, neuromotor conditions, vision and hearing impairment, speech and language deficits, seizure disorders, and behavioral problems after a 12-year follow-up (Grimwood, 2001). Subsequent research has revealed that postmeningitic children were more than twice as likely as their noninfected peers to require special educational assistance. Executive functioning skills also lagged, as they took longer to complete tasks, made more errors, were less organized, and struggled with problem-solving situations within both verbal and spatial domains (Anderson, Anderson, Grimwood, & Nolan, 2004). These findings emphasize that age at illness continues to be an important factor for long-term outcome. Children contracting meningitis at a younger age (prior to 12 months) perform more poorly on intellectual and academic evaluations and showed greatest difficulties in verbal comprehension and reading ability. Younger age at illness appears to be particularly relevant for linguistic as well as executive functions, including attentional control, planning, and reasoning, as these develop rapidly in infancy and early childhood (Anderson et al.).

Research also indicates that general health perceptions, emotions, and self-esteem in postmeningitic children without severe effects were decreased in comparison to those characteristics of a reference population of schoolchildren. Postmeningitic children with academic and/or behavior limitations manifested a clinically relevant decrease in health-related quality of life, importantly with regard to psychosocial health, cognition, and family life. Researchers found that "behavioral limitations had a more profound negative impact on quality of life than academic limitations and that children with combined limitations, both academic and behavioral, experienced the most extensive negative impact on health-related quality of life" (Koomen et al., 2005, p. 1570). Another study examined the effects of meningitis in infancy on subsequent teenage behavior and found that children who suffered from the disease during the first year of life had significantly more behavioral problems (Halket, de Louvois, Holt, & Harvey, 2003). Behavior problems were also reported as being more pronounced in a follow-up study among children who had contracted neonatal meningitis (de Louvois, Halket, & Harvey, 2005). Research indicates that 7% to 10% of postmeningitic survivors demonstrate severe neurodevelopmental effects and up to 20% experience educationally significant deficits (Anderson et al., 2004).

Diagnosis and Treatment

A definitive diagnosis of bacterial meningitis depends on the composition of the patient's CSF. This fluid is commonly extracted through a lumbar puncture, or spinal tap, for examination and culture. The usually clear liquid will appear cloudy in affected individuals, and analysis of the fluid will show an increased level of white blood cells, decreased level of glucose, and increased level of proteins (Phillips & Simor, 1998). Early diagnosis followed by appropriate medical treatment can greatly influence the course and outcome of the condition. Another diagnostic technique called Gram staining isolates the particular bacterium that is causing the meningitis, thereby determining the specific antibiotic treatment (Weir, 2002). A computed tomography (CT) scan of the head can also be helpful in assessing the degree of cranial edema, necrosis, or any displacement of brain tissue. Another technique uses a broad range of bacterial primers to detect a microbial DNA in the CSF (Sáez-Llorens & McCracken, 2003).

Patients are immediately started on antibiotic therapy and kept in respiratory isolation for 24 hours, after which they are typically noninfectious (Weir, 2002). Antibiotics decrease the number of infecting bacteria or inhibit their further growth, but the body's immune system must still eliminate the bacteria. Patients with decreased immune functioning due to HIV or AIDS, alcoholism, diabetes, malnutrition, or older age may need higher doses and more prolonged treatment to remove all bacteria (Michael, 2002).

Epidemiology, Immunization, and Prevention

Bacteria that cause meningitis regularly live in the body, most often in the nose and throat, without causing illness. Many people carrying the bacteria may never get sick yet may pass it to others. Meningitis only develops when the bacteria enters the bloodstream and travels to the CSF or the tissues that surround the brain and spinal cord. Meningococcal bacteria can spread between persons through everyday activities, including sharing drinks or kissing. Certain activities can put children at greater risk for the disease, including living in close quarters (e.g., college dormitories); being in crowded conditions for prolonged periods of time; kissing;

sharing drinking glasses, eating utensils, or water bottles; smoking or being exposed to smoke; and activities that run down and weaken the immune system, such as staying out late and having irregular sleeping patterns. Bacteria are not spread by casual contact, and meningitis is not as contagious as the common cold or flu.

In the past decade, three noteworthy events have changed the epidemiology and treatment of bacterial meningitis. The first was the introduction of the *Haemophilus influenzae* conjugate vaccine (Hib) into the United States and Western Europe as part of young children's routine vaccinations (Scheld, Koedel, Nathan, & Pfister, 2002). The Hib vaccine provides the immune system with antibodies for the *H. influenzae* strain, which enables individuals to fight off these bacteria if they are exposed to them. Cases of *H. influenzae* meningitis, once the most common type, have declined by 90% since the emergence of the Hib vaccine in 1990. The Hib vaccine has also increased the median age of onset from 9 months to 25 years within the U.S. population (Scheld et al.).

Within the United States, two kinds of meningococcal vaccines are available. They include meningococcal conjugate vaccine (MCV4) and meningococcal polysaccharide vaccine (MPSV4). Although both vaccines can prevent four types of meningococcal disease, due to its lower cost and lower incidence of side effects, MCV4 is the preferred vaccine for children and is recommended at their routine preadolescent visit (at 11 to 12 years of age).

Even though strides have been made in the past decade in preventing and treating bacterial meningitis, additional study and experimentation is needed. Today's most prolific and deadly strands of bacterial meningitis cannot be prevented through vaccination. The best preventative strategies currently offered by the medical community are to avoid contact with known infected individuals and to wash hands often and thoroughly. Given that survival rates are based on the speed of diagnosis and medical care, it is paramount to recognize the symptoms discussed above and to seek immediate medical attention at their presentation. All confirmed cases of bacterial meningitis must be reported to a local medical health officer, who can ensure the proper assessment and quarantine to control potential epidemics.

IMPLICATIONS FOR EDUCATORS

Medical treatment of meningitis includes an examination of neurological functioning both during and after hospitalization, particularly for acute neurological effects such as hydrocephalus, visual loss, hearing loss, and cerebral palsy. However, many of the known neuropsychological effects of meningitis do not become apparent until after discharge or after the discontinuation of follow-up visits (Anderson & Taylor, 2000). Prevalence rates indicate that 25% to 30% of postmeningitic survivors have significant sensory, learning, and behavioral problems, which may surface months or years later (Grimwood et al., 1995; Koomen, Grobbee, Jennekens-Schinkel, Roord, & van Furth, 2003). For example, research has indicated that teachers need to monitor postmeningitic children carefully as they reintegrate into school following hospitalization, and this monitoring should continue well into their school-age years.

An important area for follow-up monitoring is hearing loss. Researchers have found that 7% to 10% of postmeningitic children suffer a hearing loss (Berg, Trollfors, Hugosson, Fernell, & Svensson, 2002; Koomen, Grobbee, Roord, et al., 2003). In addition to hearing loss, postmeningitic survivors are more likely to exhibit poorer verbal abilities, auditory perception problems, and auditory discrimination difficulties (Anderson, Bond, Catroppa, & Grimwood, 1997; Anderson & Taylor, 2000; Grimwood et al., 1995). These auditory difficulties, if unidentified, can lead to subsequent learning and academic problems, such as reading or language-learning disabilities.

Postmeningitic children may also experience deficits in visual-motor coordination; balance and coordination problems; lower IQ scores and depressed higher-order cognitive functioning; and underachievement, grade retention, and referral to special education (Anderson & Taylor, 2000; Berg et al., 2002; Grimwood et al., 1995; Koomen, Grobbee, Jennekens-Schinkel et al., 2003). Behavioral problems have also been noted, particularly difficulties with inattention, hyperactivity, and impulsivity. Finally, more than half of post-meningitic children have been found to have subsequent general health problems, which may lead to significant school absences and therefore reduced learning opportunities (Koomen, Grobbee, Jennekens-Schinkel et al., 2003).

Educators are encouraged to develop an understanding of meningitis to provide appropriate physical and psychological support to the child. Because the disease affects each person differently, individualized treatment is necessary. Educators will need to consider issues such as school hours, communication with parents and health care providers, and the use of specialized equipment or extra help with lessons when supporting a student's return to school. Children may likely feel anxious about re-entering the school environment and present concerns about coping with day-to-day demands. A reduced school day and time for hospital and therapy appointments must be considered. It is also important that teachers remain in contact with the school psychologist and administration regarding the student's progress, with additional assessments conducted as needed to pinpoint exacerbating neuropsychological effects. Contact should also be maintained with families, as parents may report learning or behavioral problems observed at home, including problems in concentration, erratic behavior, and labile mood. Facilitating communication among all parties involved is essential in managing and supporting students who have suffered from meningitis.

EDUCATIONAL STRATEGIES

- Educate teachers, parents, and school faculty about bacterial meningitis, including its symptoms and possible aftereffects.
- Each person is affected by meningitis differently and will need to be treated individually. Accommodations to help a student to overcome the effects of the illness may include a shortened school day; technological assistance in the classroom; and maintaining communication with the student, parents, and school staff.

- Encourage all families in the school community to obtain vaccinations for meningitis.
- If a school is confronted with the death of a student following meningitis, it is important to acknowledge feelings associated with loss. Further, students will likely have many questions about the transmission of the disease and may be fearful of contamination. It is important to assure children that the organisms that cause meningitis are regularly found in our bodies and do not cause infections. School psychologists and counselors should extend their support and services to help children cope with the loss.
- Identify appropriate referral sources for families of affected students.

DISCUSSION QUESTIONS

1. How can educators, including teachers, psychologists, and administrators, support children and their families who have faced this disease?

2. What information should physicians, school psychologists, and teachers share with one another in addressing the needs of post-meningitic students?

3. Should educators encourage families to obtain the meningococcal vaccine? What are the potential risks/benefits of doing so?

4. Do schools have an obligation to ensure all students are vaccinated so as to not put the school population at risk? Should schools with dormitories require these vaccinations because of the close living quarters?

5. What must educators do to address bacterial meningitis within the school environment? What services, if any, can be offered in helping students and staff to understand the disease?

RESEARCH SUMMARY

- It is estimated that 10% to 15% of all bacterial meningitis cases are fatal and that 10% to 15% of survivors have long-term neurological damage, such as permanent hearing loss. Over 25% of survivors have significant neuropsychological effects, including sensorineural, learning, and behavioral problems.
- Meningitis vaccinations, an important prevention measure, are offered as part of routine childhood immunization schedules and recommended by the Centers for Disease Control and Prevention. It is important that parents discuss vaccinations with their child's physician. Children should also be taught good hygiene practices, such as regular hand washing and avoiding sharing of eating and drinking implements, to reduce risk of infection.
- Research on bacterial meningitis indicates that students who have suffered from the disease may present with learning disabilities, neuromotor conditions, hearing impairment, speech and language

deficits, seizure disorders, and behavioral problems. They may also demonstrate problems with executive functioning, including planning, reasoning, and goal setting.

- Students who have suffered from bacterial meningitis are more than twice as likely as their noninfected peers to require special education assistance. They are also more likely to report pessimistic perceptions about their general health, depressed emotions, and diminished self-esteem.
- The age of onset of bacterial meningitis continues to be an important factor for long-term outcome. Studies have shown that children who contract the disease prior to 12 months old perform more poorly on intellectual and academic evaluations, with greatest difficulties in verbal comprehension and reading ability.

RESOURCES

Centers for Disease Control and Prevention: www.cdc.gov/meningitis/index.html. In-depth information and resources about bacterial meningitis, including access to vaccination information.

Immunization Action Coalition: www.vaccineinformation.org/menin/. Information about bacterial meningitis, including pictures, recommendations, and links to other useful resources.

National Meningitis Association: www.nmaus.org. In-depth information about bacterial meningitis and prevention approaches.

HANDOUT

INFORMATION ABOUT BACTERIAL MENINGITIS

Meningitis is a condition in which the meninges, which are protective membranes surrounding the brain and spinal cord, become infected and inflamed, causing a complex series of neurological effects. The disease is associated with comparatively high rates of morbidity, as well as long-term neurological effects.

Because symptoms progress rapidly, parents and educators must be attentive to the early signs of infection to avoid delay in seeking medical care:

- Leg pain
- Cold hands and feet
- Abnormal skin color

The first signs of meningitis can develop quickly after a child has had a cold and runny nose, diarrhea, and vomiting or other signs of an infection. Common symptoms may include these:

- Fever
- Lethargy
- Behavioral changes
- Arching of the back
- Refusal of food
- Vomiting
- A bulging fontanel or "soft spot" at the top/front of your child's head
- Seizures
- Hemorrhagic rash, which is deep red or purple and does not fade under pressure

It is important that educators are familiar with the signs of bacterial meningitis and understand how they can support the child in the school environment. The disease has been documented to impact the cognitive, behavioral, and emotional functioning of children, particularly when endured at a younger age. Because the residual effects of bacterial meningitis vary, children may demonstrate a variety of short- and long-term effects. These can range from more debilitating effects, including deafness and brain damage, to less debilitating but still serious effects, including memory loss, distractibility, mood changes, aggression, anxiety, and depression.

10

Lyme Disease and Tick-Borne Infections*

Causes and Physical and Neuropsychological Effects in Children

Ron Hamlen and Deborah S. Kliman

Caroline's parents brought her to a psychologist because, rather suddenly, she was presenting with a variety of behaviors unusual for her. Caroline, aged 9, had always been an excellent student, cooperative, and eager to learn. She was rather shy and serious in manner, and her passions were reading and horseback riding.

Within the month previous to her first session with the psychologist, Caroline's interest in all things related to school had waned dramatically. She often asked if she could stay home. She seemed generally lethargic and no longer showed much interest in reading, taking trips to the library, or playing with her friends. Perhaps most alarming to her parents was Caroline's refusal to continue her riding lessons. She was frequently distractible or "off in her own world," both at home and in school, and was often found napping in her room.

Caroline was also demonstrating increasingly anxious behaviors. For example, she worried that something bad would happen to her parents, worried that her friends did not want to play with her, stated that her teachers did not like her anymore, and expressed fear she would be hurt while riding. None of these had ever been her concerns previously.

(Continued)

*Adapted from Hamlen, R. A., & Kliman, D. S. (2007) Lyme Disease: Etiology, neuropsychological sequelae, and educational impact. *Communiqué, 35*(5), 34–36. Copyright by the National Association of School Psychologists, Bethesda, MD. Use is by permission of the publisher. www.nasponline.org

(Continued)

She had undergone a complete physical examination, including some blood work, and her pediatrician could find nothing amiss. Her psychologist suggested a trial of antidepressant medication, but Caroline's parents were reluctant to go this route.

Caroline's parents were at a loss to think of any triggering incident that might have prompted the behaviors described. Is this young girl depressed? Suffering from an anxiety disorder? Or is there an as yet undiagnosed organic cause? What clues in Caroline's presentation might have led an educator to suspect Lyme disease and/or an associated tick-borne infection? If blood tests do not confirm a diagnosis of a tick-borne disease, then what would be the most appropriate course of action and treatment? Assuming that Caroline does have a tick-borne disease, what do her teachers and other school support personnel need to know, and how can they best support Caroline and her parents during her course of treatment?

INTRODUCTION

Education publications contain few articles on the impact of Lyme disease and associated tick-borne infections on the capacity of school-aged children to function successfully within an educational program. This oversight is of considerable concern, as educators are front-line service providers for children and adolescents presenting with symptoms of behavioral, cognitive, learning, and/or psychological problems. Educators can play a significant role in recognizing impaired school performance due to Lyme disease or other tick-borne infections and advocate for the child within the medical/school community.

BACKGROUND

Lyme disease (LD) and associated tick-borne infections (TBIs) are multisystem diseases caused by the following bacteria: *Borrelia burgdorferi* (Lyme disease spirochete), *Ehrlichia* and *Anaplasma* species (rickettsial bacteria), *Bartonella* species (bacterium), *Mycoplasma* species (bacterium), Southern tick-associated rash illness (STARI; a spirochete), and *Babesia* species (a protozoan parasite). These infectious microorganisms are generally transmitted to children from rodents or small mammals by the attachment and feeding of a deer tick or a lone star tick. The nymphal tick, whose attachment is responsible for causing the majority of infections, is the size of a poppy seed and often goes unnoticed.

The initial indications of LD infection can include but are not limited to a reddish rash, flulike illness (fever and chills), fatigue, joint pain, headache, stiff neck, mental confusion, and sleep disturbance. A single tick may transmit several of these microorganisms in the same attachment, and several of the coinfections may present with symptoms similar to those of LD. Although the risk of coinfection differs by geographic location, every tick attachment has the potential of transmitting multiple infections (Swanson, Neitzel, Reed, & Belongia, 2006). In addition, the LD spirochete possesses molecular survival strategies, enabling it to evade the immune response and to persist in its human host (Rupprecht, Koedel, Fingerle, & Pfister, 2008). Misdiagnosis and delayed treatment frequently lead to debilitating chronic illness with relapses and deterioration, especially in musculoskeletal, cognitive, and neuropsychiatric impairments (Fallon, Kochevar, Gaito, & Nields, 1998; Halperin, 2004). Symptoms often have puzzling presentation in patients, especially in children (Fallon et al.).

Although some school nurses are alert to the impact of LD and associated TBIs on school-aged children (e.g., Healy, 2000), information on these diseases is generally absent from the education and psychology literature. Educators require a basic understanding of the diagnosis and treatment of TBIs. They must also be able to recognize and articulate the impaired school performance frequently caused by these illnesses and advocate for the student with illness within the school, family, and medical communities.

Infection Incidence and Risk

Lyme disease is the fastest-growing vector-transmitted disease in the United States, with a 38% increase in the Centers for Disease Control surveillance cases from 2006 to 2007 (CDC, 2007; 2008). Roughly 20,000 new cases of LD are diagnosed each year, and the CDC (2007) acknowledges underreporting. This is particularly troublesome because of the incidence of pediatric cases (Young, 1998).

Lyme disease is endemic in the Northeastern and mid-Atlantic states, in the upper North-Central region, and in northern California. Twelve states—Connecticut, Delaware, Maine, Maryland, Massachusetts, Minnesota, New Hampshire, New Jersey, New York, Pennsylvania, Rhode Island, and Wisconsin—account for 95% of cases reported nationally (CDC, 2007). Lyme disease has been documented in every state, and associated TBIs are reported in the same geographical areas as LD.

People of all ages are vulnerable to LD, and significant infection rates occur in children aged 5 to 14 years (CDC, 2007). Children in suburban residential areas surrounded by tick-infested woods and those who participate in outdoor recreational activities are at the greatest risk of getting LD or other TBIs. Infection can occur from childhood activities in a shady home environment, especially where ground cover, moist humus, and leaf litter dominate play areas (Klein, Eppes, & Hunt, 1996). Each spring, the risk of infection increases significantly; as temperatures reach 40°F (4.5°C), ticks become active, and outdoor activities increase (Lane, Steinlein, & Mun, 2004). Although every tick might not be infected, every tick attachment has the potential for transmitting LD and associated TBIs.

Diagnosis

The central diagnostic difficulty responsible for the current debate within the medical community on diagnosis and treatment of LD and TBIs is the lack of definitive and readily available laboratory tests for active infection (Coulter et al., 2005). Physicians are challenged to diagnose early TBIs based on clinical presentations (patient history, exposure risk, and symptoms). Laboratory test data, including those for coinfections, can be supportive in diagnosis (Sherr, 2004). The Food and Drug Administration (FDA; Brown, Hansen, Langone, Lowe, & Pressly, 1999) has questioned the reliability of commonly marketed LD test kits and stated that they "should **never** be the primary basis for making diagnostic or treatment decisions" (p. 1). The CDC (2007) has commented that test data based on CDC LD surveillance case definition, as reported with the test kits, is not to be used in diagnosis and treatment decisions. Both the CDC and FDA have acknowledged that a clinical diagnosis is the "best practice." No test can rule out the possibility of infection (Coulter et al., 2005). School psychologists and nurses, educators, pediatricians, and primary care physicians need to be aware of the occurrence rates, potential severity, and diagnostic dilemmas of all TBIs. With our mobile society, this is true in both TBI-endemic and nonendemic areas.

Neurological and Cognitive Deficits

Lyme disease is characterized by a strong pro-inflammatory response, which can involve the brain, and an aberrant innate pro-inflammatory response, which is involved in chronic illness (Rupprecht et al., 2008). Cognitive symptoms are a direct result of dysfunction of the cerebral cortex where cognitive processing occurs (Bransfield, Brand, & Sherr, 2001). Although children with LD and TBIs can experience a variety of symptoms, it is often the subtle neurological and cognitive deficits, which may elude detection, that have the most negative effect on a child's school performance and social life. Children with multiple TBIs frequently present with more diverse and severe symptoms compared to children with LD alone (Swanson et al., 2006).

These symptoms should be red flags for unrecognized LD and associated TBIs:

- Headache (can be severe), neck stiffness
- Peripheral neuropathy (nerve pain) in back, legs, or hands; musculoskeletal pain (can be severe)
- Distal paresthesia (tingling sensation, often in legs and hands) and facial paralysis
- Deficits with short-term memory, including with sequential, spatial, and tracking tasks; slowed word and name retrieval, letter and number reversals
- Decreased reading comprehension and handwriting skills
- Impaired speech fluency, including stuttering and slurred speech
- Inability to perform accurately previously mastered mathematical calculations
- Vision problems, including difficulty in the classroom in seeing and following visually presented material, frequent blinking or tics, inability to coordinate eye movement, and targeting difficulties
- Movement and coordination impairment, balance problems, clumsiness, or vertigo
- Executive function impairment, including the inability to activate or sustain effort and attention or manage frustration, confusion and lethargic thinking, and difficulty expressing thoughts

- Frequent errors in speaking, writing, spelling; dyslexic-like behaviors
- Severe and chronic fatigue unrelieved by rest, which may be evidenced by falling asleep in class; missing class because of sleep disturbance and/or sporadic night sweats
- Emotional and uncharacteristic behavioral presentation, including withdrawal from peers or a shift to a lower-functioning group, depersonalization (loss of a sense of physical existence), cessation of involvement in sports or other extracurricular activities, inattentiveness, attention deficit behavior, obsessive-compulsiveness, depression, anxiety, panic, aggression, defiance, explosive outbursts, mood swings, irritability, hyperactivity, nightmares, and sudden suicidal thoughts
- Inability to perform at grade level, which may be evidenced as inconsistent or sloppy schoolwork, late assignments, lower grades, feeling overwhelmed by schoolwork, missed school days, and school phobia
- Other neurological manifestations, including tinnitus, trigeminal neuralgia, facial numbness, sensory hyperacusis (unusual sensitivity to sound), photophobia, and intrusive and distorted visual images

Every child with LD or TBIs has a unique symptom profile that varies significantly during the process of infection. In addition to declining cognitive ability and declining school performance, additional presenting physical symptoms include gastrointestional manifestations, such as chronic abdominal pain, gastritis, duodenitis, and colitis (Fried, Abel, Pietrucha, Kuo, & Bal, 1999); and cardiac complications, such as irregular rhythm, carditis, and heart block (Chen, 2008). In addition, ocular symptoms, including optic neuritis, neuropathy, conjunctivitis, uveitis, keratitis, ocular pain, or vision loss, are common (Rothermel, Hedges, & Steere, 2001).

Developmental Delay, Attention Disorders, and Autism Spectrum Disorders

Clinical experience suggests that in a subset of pediatric patients, LD and TBIs can mimic developmental delay and autism spectrum disorders (Bransfield, Wulfman, Harvey, & Ysman, 2008; Bransfield, 2009; Nicolson, 2007). Cognitive and behavioral difficulties are also similar to those observed in affective, oppositional defiant, and attention deficit disorders (Tager et al., 2001). Infection can also exacerbate pre-existing behavioral or psychiatric illness (Bransfield, 2007).

Depressive, Panic, and Aggressive Disorders

Rarely are children initially diagnosed with psychiatric manifestations of LD or TBIs, because their complaints are vague and thought to be functional in nature. If the undiagnosed disease process has psychiatric manifestations that lower the child's frustration tolerance and/or increase irritability and impair cognitive functioning, then a referral from the school or treating physician to a psychiatrist addressing the assumed psychogenic or functional disorder is likely (Bransfield, 2007). Although much of the data on psychiatric illness in children due to LD and TBIs is anecdotal, 60% of confirmed LD adult patients reported an episode of major depression during their illness (Rachman & Garfield, 1998). Moreover, significant numbers of hospitalized psychiatric patients were found seropositive for *B. burgdorferi* relative to healthy comparison subjects (Hajek et al., 2002). Clinical experience suggests a link between TBIs and aggression in children and adolescents (Bransfield, 2001).

Long-Term Outcomes

When facial nerve palsy was the initial symptom of LD and appropriately treated with antibiotics, neuropsychological and cognitive functioning and general health outcomes (based on neuropsychologic tests) were comparable to those in patients who did not have LD (Vazquez, Sparrow, & Shapiro, 2003). With initial dermatological or neurological symptoms, studies also indicated significant recovery (Adams, Rose, Eppes, & Klein, 1999). However, Bloom, Wyckoff, Meissner, and Steere (1998) reported that in patients with late neurologic manifestations of LD, improvement was often gradual or with continuing multiple neurocognitive symptoms requiring IV antibiotics. Adolescents with a history of treated LD can be at risk for long-term problems in cognition and school functioning (McAuliffe, Brassard, & Fallon, 2008).

IMPLICATIONS FOR EDUCATORS

Educators address few phenomena that are as emotionally and clinically challenging as diagnosing the cause of a child's cognitive deterioration (Shaw, 2005). When pediatric TBIs are diagnosed early and treated promptly, few children develop long-term cognitive deficits (Vazquez et al., 2003) or require significant educational services. However, some children remain ill even after appropriate treatment (Berenbaum, 2004; Bransfield et al., 2001; McAuliffe et al., 2008). Often these children have had symptoms for months or years and been seen by several physicians who have erroneously labeled the child hypochondriac, psychosomatic, depressed, or malingering (Healy, 2000). The school psychologist and educator should perceive the symptoms as red flags when conducting intelligence testing, curriculum-based assessments, and direct student observation. Educators should play a multifaceted role in the identification of this illness by interviewing parents, as well as teachers or child care workers from previous years, to compare past with current performance. In addition, the school psychologist can be a postdiagnosis student advocate and active participant in the school and community medical management of the student's illness. Follow-up skill assessment to provide discrete data to audit the effects of educational accommodation and progress of medical treatment is necessary.

Section 504 of the Rehabilitation Act of 1973, the Americans with Disabilities Act (ADA) of 1990, and the 2004 Individuals with Disabilities Education Act (IDEA) mandate that students with disabilities in elementary, secondary, and postsecondary schools receiving federal financial assistance cannot be discriminated against because of their disabilities. In many cases, schools are required to provide accommodations and/or supportive individual educational programs to help ill students achieve their academic goals (Betz, 2001). Accommodations include shortened days, untimed tests, the dropping of unnecessary requirements, alternative testing methods, separate/quieter testing locations, and modified home instruction programs (Msall et al., 2003).

IDEA obliges school districts to identify disabled and potentially disabled children and refer them to a Child Study Team, on which the school psychologist is an active member, to develop an Individualized Educational Program (IEP), monitor the IEP, and revise the IEP as needed (Boyce, Gelfman, & Schwab, 2000). Children with Lyme disease or TBIs should lead as full and normal a life as possible, given the severity of their illness. They are covered under Section 504, ADA, and IDEA legislation.

Because educational personnel may not be familiar with the physical, neurological, and emotional ramifications of LD or associated TBIs in the school setting, the school psychologist, in cooperation with the school nurse and special education teacher, can provide insight about the illness and needed educational accommodations (Cavendish, 2003).

Whenever a change in a child's behavior, mood, or overall functioning occurs, including a suspected attention deficit/hyperactivity disorder, LD or TBIs should be considered quickly, as delays in diagnosis are associated with chronicity and morbidity (Fallon et al., 1998). Children and adolescents with LD who display considerable impairment and whose diagnosis and treatment are delayed have significantly more school-related cognitive and psychiatric sequelae than healthy children (McAuliffe et al., 2008; Tager et al., 2001). School psychologists, educators, nurses, and teachers may be the first adults with an opportunity to recognize the possible underlying infectious origin of presenting symptoms.

Effects of LD and TBI include fatigue, school tardiness, memory problems, distractibility, attention difficulties, and inability to understand complex information. These children also have behavioral disorders (e.g., irritability, anxiety, and depression) and school performance deterioration. Less is known about the long-term outcome for children with coinfections, as less research has been published. Clinical experience suggests that when the coinfections are effectively treated before treating LD, the outcome is favorable. Untreated coinfections, however, can lead to chronic illness, often involving severe neurological and cognitive problems.

EDUCATIONAL STRATEGIES

- Communicate with parents and, with appropriate permission, medical professionals concerning the child's medical status. Educators can provide important information to physicians and parents on changes in academic performance, social and emotional functioning, and eating habits.

- Being flexible with assignments is critical. Children with LD or TBIs often have fluctuating levels of attention and alertness.
- Plans for itinerate homebound instruction may be necessary when children are not able to attend school.
- Allowing additional time for assignments may be necessary.
- Other strategies include shortened days, untimed tests, the dropping of unnecessary requirements, alternative testing methods, separate/quieter testing locations, and modified home instruction programs

DISCUSSION QUESTIONS

1. What features are common to presentations of uncharacteristic behavioral and cognitive symptoms in school-aged children with Lyme disease or other tick-borne infections?

2. Are tick-borne diseases endemic, common, or rare in your location?

3. Why might blood and laboratory tests be unreliable in detecting tick-borne diseases?

4. Why might it be difficult to distinguish the symptoms of a tick-borne illness from behavioral and cognitive symptoms from other causes?

5. What other commonly diagnosed conditions may present symptoms similar to those of a tick-borne illness?

6. What consequences does delayed treatment have for children with a tick-borne illness?

RESEARCH SUMMARY

- Lyme disease and tick-borne diseases are common and often under-diagnosed.
- Lyme disease and tick-borne diseases have widely varied symptoms, including changes in cognitive and behavioral functioning.
- There are no clear laboratory tests for the diagnosis of Lyme and tick-based diseases. The diagnosis is made clinically on the basis of presenting symptoms.
- Several medical conditions have clinical symptoms similar to those of Lyme disease, making diagnosis extremely difficult.
- Treatment for Lyme disease can be challenging. The organism causing Lyme disease can lie dormant and then become active again at a later time. However, when treatment is effective, cognitive functioning, health status, and emotional functioning often return to pre-infection levels.

RESOURCES

Hamlen R. A., & Kliman D. S. (2007). Lyme disease: Etiology, neuropsychological sequelae, and educational impacts. *Communiqué, 35*, 34–36.
Lang, D. (1997). *Coping with Lyme disease* (2nd ed.). New York: Henry Holt.

HANDOUT

PEDIATRIC LYME DISEASE AND ASSOCIATED TICK-BORNE INFECTIONS

Whenever a change in a child's behavior, mood, or overall functioning occurs, including a suspected attention deficit/hyperactivity disorder, Lyme disease (LD) or tick-borne infections (TBIs) should be considered quickly as delays in diagnosis are associated with chronic impairment. Parents and educators need to be aware of the possibility of LD and TBIs as they may be first to recognize the possible underlying infectious origin of aberrant student behavior. Lyme disease and TBIs have become a permanent part of America's public health landscape, affecting most perilously its young, their families, and school community. Many children seriously affected by these infections have alterations in personality, cognitive functioning, and behavior.

Infection Incidence and Risk

- Lyme disease is the fastest growing vector-transmitted disease in the United States with about 20,000 new cases reported each year.
- Lyme disease occurs nationwide; however, twelve states—Connecticut, Delaware, Maine, Maryland, Massachusetts, Minnesota, New Hampshire, New Jersey, New York, Pennsylvania, Rhode Island, and Wisconsin—account for 95% of cases reported.
- People of all ages are vulnerable to LD, yet significant infection rates occur in school-aged children.
- Children in endemic suburban residential areas surrounded by tick-infested woods and those who participate in outdoor recreational activities are at risk of getting LD and associated TBIs. Even the city child on a nature outing is at risk with the greatest potential for infection in the spring.

Overview of Diseases

Lyme disease and TBIs are multi-system bacterial and protozoan diseases. These disease-causing microorganisms are transmitted to humans from rodents or small mammals through the attachment and feeding of a deer tick or a lone star tick. A single tick may co-transmit several of these microorganisms in the same attachment, which is often unnoticed due to the small, poppy seed-sized tick. Initial indications of infection can include but are not limited to a reddish rash, flu-like symptoms (fever, chills), fatigue, joint pain, headache, stiff neck, mental confusion, and sleeping disturbance. Symptoms are complex and often have puzzling presentations in children. An individual can have LD and TBIs repeatedly.

Diagnosis

Physicians are challenged to diagnose early TBIs based on clinical presentations (patient history, exposure risk, and symptoms). Laboratory test data are of limited reliability, identifying only about 50% of infections. A large body of clinical evidence illustrates that diagnosis of LD is especially difficult when the rash is absent, laboratory tests are negative, uncharacteristic symptoms occur (based on physician experience), and/or atypical psychiatric symptoms are present. The task of separating a primary pediatric psychiatric disorder from psychiatric LD and certain TBIs can be daunting and brain imaging technologies and psychological testing may be required. Misdiagnosis and delayed treatment of TBIs frequently lead to debilitating chronic illness and cognitive impairments.

School Performance

Every child with LD or TBIs has a unique profile of symptoms, which can vary significantly during the process of infection. Although children with TBIs can experience a plethora of symptoms, it is often the subtle multiple cognitive and neurologic deficits that elude prior detection. These deficits have the most profound negative impact on a child's school performance and social life.

Frequently symptoms develop in a child who previously performed well within the school environment. A challenging manifestation of TBIs is that symptoms may persist or they may be episodic and fluctuating in type and severity, further confusing diagnosis. Based on teacher or parental observations, the child may not appear sick in the traditional sense. Disease onset can be gradual with increasing fatigue, social disinterest, or deteriorating school performance. An important finding is that multiple cognitive and behavioral difficulties are similar to those observed with affective, oppositional defiant, attention deficit, and possible autism spectrum disorders. Further complicating diagnosis is the inability of children and teenagers to express their feelings to parents, teachers or friends.

Children are not initially diagnosed with psychiatric manifestations of TBIs because their complaints are seen as vague and inconsequential. If the undiagnosed disease has psychiatric manifestations, then a referral from the school or treating physician to a psychiatrist is likely.

What Can Parents and Educators Do?

- The most important action for parents is to prevent infection. Many universities and public health departments can provide information on tick repellants, protective clothing, high risk areas and behaviors to avoid, landscape chemical applications, and tick control on pets.
- However, if symptoms and school problems occur due to LD or other TBIs, it is imperative that parents and teachers collaborate, in consultation with a school psychologist and/or nurse to take appropriate medical intervention. Effective parent/teacher communication is crucial to discuss events in the home and school life, the problems they encounter, and feelings that result. It is vital for the parents and school to monitor the ill child's behavior, assessing positive and negative changes, and communicating these observations.
- Parents and educators can be post-diagnosis advocates and active participants in seeking necessary school accommodations. Frequently, children with LD or associated TBIs and who struggle to remain in school hear comments from their classmates (often behind their back) about their "drama" and that they are just faking for attention. This experience can be devastating to the child's emotional stability and parents and teachers need to support the child and raise awareness in the school community.
- Federal law, that is, Section 504 of the Federal Rehabilitation Act of 1973, the Americans with Disabilities Act (ADA) of 2000, and the 2004 Individuals with Disabilities Education Act (IDEA), mandates that students with disabilities in elementary, secondary, and post-secondary schools receiving federal financial assistance not be discriminated against because of their disabilities. In many cases, schools are required to provide needed accommodations and/or supportive Individualized Educational Programs (IEPs).
- Accommodations include shortened days, un-timed tests, dropping unnecessary requirements, alternative testing methods, separate/quieter testing locations, and modified home instruction programs. Children with Lyme disease should lead as full and normal a life as they are capable of given the severity of their illness.

Prevention and Wellness Intervention

11

Childhood Obesity Prevention*

A Review for Educators

Jessica A. Hoffman and Laura Anderson

Northside Elementary School is located in a large, urban school district. Over 50% of the students are Latino, and 30% are African-American. Data from the school nurse indicate that 45% of the students are either overweight (BMI-for-age = 85%–94.9%) or obese (BMI-for-age > 95). In 2006, the school district developed a wellness policy that prohibits the sale of sugar-sweetened beverages, has guidelines regulating the types of foods that can be sold on school grounds, prohibits candy and bake sales as fundraisers, and requires that students receive at least 90 hours of physical education per school year in addition to nutrition education as part of their general education curriculum. Individual schools in the district are responsible for ensuring the wellness policy is implemented, and principals are required to document specific, measurable ways in which their buildings adhere to the policy.

Northside has many competing educational initiatives that staff must attend to; however, both school staff and parents believe children's physical health is critically important for learning and that school should be a place where children can have opportunities to be physically active and to eat well. Even before the wellness policy was adopted, Northside had a number of initiatives in place to help children to be physically active. Although the school does not have funds in its budget for a physical education teacher, which makes it impossible for the school to meet the district's physical education requirement, the school has a relationship with a local

*Adapted from Blom-Hoffman, J. (2004). Obesity prevention in children: Strategies for parents and school personnel. *Communiqué, 33*(3), `Insert'. Copyright by the National Association of School Psychologists, Bethesda, MD. Use is by permission of the publisher. www.nasponline.org

community center, so students receive swimming instruction during school. Also, the school has a well-coordinated, structured recess program. As such, students are physically active on the playground, and fights are kept to a minimum. Finally, the school houses several afterschool programs that provide opportunities for students to be physically active free of charge.

Although it is required, Northside does not have formal, structured health education as part of the curriculum. Also, bake sales and candy sales are frequent occurrences. Most students participate in the free lunch program; however, according to students and staff, the school lunch is in desperate need of improvement. Teachers frequently witness students take a lunch tray from the lunch line, proceed directly to the garbage, throw out everything except the milk, and then purchase a bag of cookies.

Consider the following: How can teachers, administrators, and parents work together to improve the quality of food served in the school meals program? How can the building principal obtain funding for a physical education program? How can school staff address students' health needs related to healthy eating and physical activity, given their need to focus on students' academic success as measured in the statewide testing program? What are the long-term consequences of a poor nutritional environment and few opportunities for physical activity for children in school?

INTRODUCTION

The rates of overweight and obesity in children and adolescents have risen dramatically since the 1970s. Nationally, nearly one in three school-aged children is overweight or obese (Ogden, Carroll, & Flegal, 2008). These rates are even higher in certain minority groups, with disproportionately higher rates among Hispanic and African-American children and adolescents compared with their non-Hispanic White peers (Ogden et al.). Excess body weight is a problem because it is related to many serious medical and social problems, including Type 2 diabetes, heart disease, high blood pressure, stroke, sleep apnea, some cancers, depression, low self-esteem, and social isolation (U.S. Department of Health and Human Services, 2001). The causes of childhood obesity are multifaceted, but educators can play an important role in promoting children's healthy eating and physical activity at school and at home.

BACKGROUND

A world of metabolically identical individuals in equivalent environments would render the prevention of pediatric overweight scientifically simple: We would create the ideal energy balance equation (i.e., calories in versus calories out). However, several recent meta-analyses and literature reviews have come to one notable conclusion: Pediatric obesity is a biopsychosocial condition that has not yet demonstrated a *reliable* intervention response (Adair, 2008; Doak, Visscher, Renders, & Seidell, 2006; IOM, 2007; Small, Anderson, & Melnyk, 2007; Stice, Shaw, & Marti, 2006). The evidence base highlights the need for an ecological perspective when addressing this multifaceted problem. Because pediatric obesity is associated with a number of factors that interact in complex ways, its prevention will entail multilevel, systematic collaboration across contexts.

Child and Family Context

Biological Factors. Childhood obesity has multiple biological bases. Kral and Faith (2008) examined the behavioral genetics of childhood obesity and eating patterns, reviewing over 10 years of studies that demonstrated that obesity runs in families and is heritable. Furthermore, the eating in the absence of hunger (EAH) behavioral trait has strong biological components. That is, eating in response to external (versus hunger) cues has genetic underpinnings and tends to remain relatively stable throughout life (Kral & Faith). Other researchers have identified additional biological bases of obesity, including (a) hormonal predictors such as reduced leptin and ghrelin levels, often associated with sleep deprivation, and (b) family similarities in reduced frontal cortical activity related to appetite disinhibition and dysregulated satiety cues (Adair, 2008; Kral & Faith; Riggs, Kobayakawa Sakuma, & Pentz, 2007).

Research examining the biological underpinnings of childhood obesity has emphasized the mismatch between a child's physiology and his or her surrounding environments (Adair, 2008; IOM, 2007). Adair emphasized different developmental periods and the obesogenic susceptibilities across the child-adolescent trajectory. For example, babies born to mothers who developed maternal gestational diabetes are more likely to be overweight. Growth rate in the first 4 months of life also predicts childhood BMI; rapid growth is associated with increased BMI. Finally, in the early adolescent period, early maturation (e.g., menarche before age 11) has been associated with increased rates of child/adolescent overweight (see Adair for further reading on this topic).

Behavioral Factors. Behavioral factors at the child, peer, and family levels comprise much of the early childhood obesity literature (IOM, 2007). Children's dietary and physical activity patterns at home and with peers contribute to their weight status. For example, if children spend large amounts of their time with peers playing sedentary video games or watching television and eating high-calorie snack foods, it is less likely that optimal energy balance will be realized. In addition, snacking between meals and ignoring hunger cues are behaviors acquired through habit (Doak et al., 2006; Riggs et al., 2007). The reinforcing value of obesity-promoting behaviors (e.g., watching television and eating foods high in fat and sugar) is often much stronger than that of traditional healthy weight behaviors (e.g., eating fresh fruits and vegetables and being physically active).

Family behaviors also impact children's weight status. In recent years, fewer children sit down to eat meals with their families, and reduced family connectedness is associated with higher rates of childhood obesity (Doak et al., 2006; Jenkins & Horner, 2005). Campbell and colleagues (2007) examined multiple aspects of the home food environment and found that behavioral factors were powerful in predicting child obesity. Parent provision of healthy food at home, modeling healthy eating behaviors, and authoritative parenting style were all associated with healthy weight and positive outcomes (Campbell et al.).

Socioeconomic and Cultural Factors at the Family Level. Lower socio-economic status (SES) is associated with increased rates of obesity (IOM, 2007; Small et al., 2007). Families with fewer economic resources typically have reduced access to affordable, healthy, varied foods, as well as to physical activities that may cost money outside of the school setting. Furthermore, some cultural food preferences may not promote energy balance, and families may have neither experience with nor knowledge of healthier cooking techniques. Also, culturally preferred healthy foods (e.g., fresh fruits, beans, vegetables) may be neither available nor affordable in local stores. It is also important to note family responses to school-delivered lifestyle change interventions. Low-income and/or ethnic minority families may perceive healthy weight programming as a negative judgment if it is not delivered in a culturally competent manner (IOM). Today's fast-paced family life has also impacted children's weight status. For example, in two-working-parent households, there is less time (or a perception of insufficient time) to prepare healthy meals (Doak et al., 2006) and low-cost, pre-prepared, processed foods (e.g., fast food) are relied upon for many family meals.

The Community

Effective obesity prevention efforts must surpass the individual and family. Evidence demonstrates the association between the community context and rates of obesity (IOM, 2007; Jenkins & Horner, 2005). The built environment (i.e., the availability of sidewalks, trails, bike paths, and parks) has an impact on physical activity, and the context surrounding the use of the built environment also matters. For example, if a neighborhood overflows with people enjoying paths and trails, others likely will feel inspired to use those trails. On the other hand, if a park or playground is located in an unsafe neighborhood, it would be unwise for parents to allow their children to play independently at that location (Jenkins & Horner). The availability and use of sidewalks and trails influences the number of children who ride bicycles to school. Finally, community athletic and country clubs promoting physical activity are selectively available. Not all communities have or can afford access to these amenities.

Financially impoverished and racially segregated communities tend to have fewer fresh, healthy foods available for purchase (Baker, Schootman, Barnidge, & Kelly, 2006; Morland & Filomena, 2007), and when available, these foods can be more costly than less healthy foods (Neault, Cook, Morris, & Frank, 2005). Convenience stores—full of packaged, high-calorie snack foods and sugar-sweetened beverages—abound in these communities (Doak et al., 2006; IOM, 2007). The feasibility and utility of energy-dense convenience foods for lower-income families make it difficult to eat healthfully.

The School

Intraschool Processes. Emerging data have revealed that the culture of schools, as well as local and/or state standards pertaining to academic achievement and physical activity, can impact students' weight status (Budd & Volpe, 2006). For example, teachers have identified time and financial resources as two key barriers to implementing healthy weight promotion programming in schools (IOM, 2007). The school day is limited, and—given current mandates—teachers must focus on academic subject matter assessed via high-stakes testing. This emphasis inherently results in fewer student opportunities for physical activity (Doak et al., 2006).

The typical length of the American school day in conjunction with curricular requirements also limits the amount of time available for school lunch periods. Jenkins and Horner (2005) found that adolescents identified the amount of time for lunch as the biggest barrier to healthy eating at school.

The social world of children and adolescents likewise interacts with intraschool processes to contribute to weight status. For example, an open campus permitting teens to exit for lunch has been identified as a barrier to improving healthy weight (IOM, 2007). School cafeterias offering appealing social environments and plenty of healthy choices may ameliorate this situation.

When describing school-based influences on healthy weight, the sociocontextual processes surrounding school athletics cannot be ignored. In schools where the athletically talented students participate in organized sports, the majority of children are left without such opportunities. An increase in intramural, club, nontraditional, and afterschool physical activity programs can address this need (Budd & Volpe, 2006; Jenkins & Horner, 2005).

Intraschool processes involving teachers and professionals can affect weight status. Modeling and reinforcement of messages supporting healthy energy balance by interventionists across the school environment is a promising practice (IOM, 2007). Furthermore, programs would have increased sustainability and buy-in if implemented by a diverse group of personnel (Budd & Volpe, 2006). Several recent studies have noted how well suited school nurses are for schoolwide health promotion. They have individual and institutional access to students, and they can be particularly supportive with family involvement (Berry, Savoye, Melkus, & Grey, 2007; Kubik, Story, & Davey, 2007; Mauriello et al., 2006).

School Environment. Several features of the school environment itself impact weight status. Food in the cafeteria is associated with reduced student BMI, for example, when a large selection of fresh produce and few to no energy-dense à la carte items are available for purchase (IOM, 2007; Jenkins & Horner, 2005). Competitive foods available through vending machines and related advertising, school stores, and fundraisers need further examination to determine their impact on childhood obesity (Budd & Volpe, 2006; Doak et al., 2006; IOM).

Finally, the built environment at school can facilitate or hinder healthy weight promotion efforts. Plentiful bicycle racks combined with bike-to-school programs, creative playgrounds with structured recess activities and sufficient adult monitoring, and schoolwide physical activity equipment may encourage increased energy expenditure. Innovative integration of physical activity in the school environment is likely advantageous, but this is one of the most critical gaps in the literature (Budd & Volpe, 2006; IOM, 2007). An essential question for educators is this: Can more engaging physical activity at school be incorporated cost-effectively while also enhancing academic outcomes (see Ratey, 2008, for more information related to this topic).

Family, Community, and School: Healthy Weight Facilitated

As evidence has surfaced regarding the synergistic effects of obesogenic environments for children, nationwide efforts have become more proactive. School wellness plans, as required by the Child Nutrition WIC Reauthorization Act of 2004 (see IOM, 2007, for further reading), have raised consciousness regarding energy balance, healthy weight in children, and the powerful potential of the school as a lifestyle change agent. Comprehensive school health programs, school-based community activity centers, and school-based health clinics have emerged as vehicles for multileveled program implementation (Adair, 2008; Budd & Volpe, 2006; Doak et al., 2006; IOM).

Although these efforts are promising, much work lies ahead when considering the number of children and adolescents classified as overweight and obese (Adair, 2008; Ogden et al., 2008). To advance school-based obesity prevention research, efforts must focus on the collection of quality data that are meaningful to stakeholders (IOM, 2007). The systematic translations of ecologically valid, evidence-based approaches will likely lead to positive outcomes.

Given the continued lack of valid and reliable interventions to prevent and treat childhood obesity, in conjunction with the host of risk factors surrounding children, innovation in prevention and intervention is required. Schools serve an important role in healthy weight promotion, given that most children spend many of their waking hours and eat multiple meals in this setting. As childhood obesity is one of the only lifestyle diseases striking our population at such a young age and in epidemic proportions, schools must capitalize on a unique ecological role: Feasible, multicomponent prevention may not be realizable elsewhere. Schools have the responsibility to enlist collaborators and to activate innovation, evaluation, and documentation of ecological obesity prevention. To date, prevention efforts have not matched the severity of the problem.

EDUCATIONAL STRATEGIES

Encouraging children to eat diets that are high in fruit, vegetables, and whole grains can be challenging due to the higher costs of these foods, the decreased availability of these foods in poorer communities, and the convenience of getting inexpensive meals at fast-food restaurants. The following ideas can help children develop healthy eating behaviors:

- Small changes, such as the type of snack foods bought, can be a good place to start to develop healthier eating behaviors. Fruit, vegetables, cheese, yogurt, and whole-grain crackers can be purchased in place of cakes, chips, doughnuts, candy, and cookies. Children can be involved in food shopping and food preparation.
- Parents are influential role models, so it is important that they make healthy eating choices around children.

- All foods can be enjoyed infrequently and in small quantities. Restricting foods only increases their value and makes children want them even more.
- Foods should not be used as a reward, as this only increases their value to a child.
- Many children are hesitant to eat foods that are new to them. Sometimes it can take 10 to 15 exposures to a new food before a young child likes it. Being persistent (but not pushy or forceful) in encouraging children to eat new foods by providing repeated exposures of small quantities can be helpful. You can ask a child to take a "no thank you" bite of the new food if she or he does not want to eat it.
- Finally, parents should ask their child's health care provider how many calories he or she should consume each day for optimal growth and development. This number will depend on the child's age, gender, and level of physical activity.

Help children be physically active and reduce sedentary activity or "screen time."

- The U.S. Department of Health and Human Services and the National Association for Sport and Physical Education recommend that school-age children and adolescents get at least 60 minutes of age-appropriate physical activity on all or most days of the week.
- Opportunities to engage in physical activity in recess and gym class should not be withheld as a punishment.
- Physical activities should be varied in nature and should occur multiple times per day, lasting at least 15 minutes per occasion. At school, physical education and structured recess programs are obvious places where children and adolescents can be active. Afterschool programs are another important place where children can be active. In addition, communities can organize Safe Routes to School programs to encourage walking and biking (see www.saferoutesinfo.org).
- Parents can advocate for expanded physical education programs at parent council meetings if their child's school district does not provide physical education multiple times per week.
- Physical activity levels tend to decline in adolescence, so it is important to find ways to motivate teens to be active.
- Too much "screen time," which includes watching television, playing video games, or using the computer, has been linked to childhood overweight. The American Academy on Pediatrics recommends that children's "screen time" be limited to no more than 1 to 2 hours per day.

DISCUSSION QUESTIONS

1. What factors contribute to childhood obesity? How do these factors relate to each other? Why is it so difficult to address this problem?
2. What can educators do to help create healthier school environments that promote healthy weight?

3. How can school staff, families, and communities work together to help children eat healthier and be more active?

4. From an ecological perspective, how do systemic factors, such as laws, policies, and industry, contribute to the obesity problem?

5. What are the long-term consequences of not preventing childhood obesity?

RESEARCH SUMMARY

- Maintaining a healthy weight is a challenge for adults and children.
- Overweight is in part due to easy access to large portions of high-calorie, low-cost foods being marketed toward children, as well as limited availability of high-quality, affordable fruits, vegetables, and whole-grain foods in many communities.
- Childhood obesity has multiple biological bases. Eating in the absence of hunger has genetic underpinnings and tends to remain relatively stable throughout life. Other biological bases of obesity include reduced leptin and ghrelin levels, often associated with sleep deprivation, and family similarities in reduced frontal cortical activity related to appetite disinhibition and dysregulated satiety cues.
- Children's dietary and physical activity patterns at home and with peers contribute to their weight status. These patterns include playing sedentary video games or watching television while eating high-calorie snack foods.
- Family behaviors also impact children's weight status. Parental provision of healthy food at home, modeling of healthy eating behaviors, and authoritative parenting style are all associated with healthy weight and positive health outcomes.
- Parents can help their children achieve a healthy weight by making sure they eat nutritiously within caloric recommendations and get appropriate physical activity.

RESOURCES

Action for Healthy Kids: www.actionforhealthykids.org. This Web site offers a variety of resources for improving nutrition and physical activity in schools and a state-by-state index of improvements currently in place.

Alliance for a Healthier Generation: www.healthiergeneration.org. The Healthy Schools Program portion of this Web site provides tools and solutions for schools to become healthier places for both students and staff, including ideas for nonfood fundraisers and food and beverage guidelines.

Centers for Disease Control and Prevention: Division of Nutrition, Physical Activity and Obesity: www.cdc.gov/nccdphp/dnpa/index.htm. This helpful Web site provides information to get started on making healthy eating and physical activity changes.

Dole Superkids: www.dolesuperkids.com. This is an engaging Web site for children to help them eat more fruits and vegetables. It also provides useful resources for parents and school personnel.

Fruits and Veggies More Matters: www.fruitsandveggiesmatter.gov. This useful Web site provides information to help meet fruit and vegetable consumption guidelines.

Healthy Schools: Healthy Youth!: www.cdc.gov/HealthyYouth/index.htm. This Web site from the Centers for Disease Control and Prevention provides helpful resources for school personnel related to nutrition and physical activity.

In addition, this article by Marion Nestle provides straightforward dietary guidance:

Nestle, M. (2007, September). Eating made simple. *Scientific American*, 60–69). Available September 19, 2009, at http://www.scientificamerican.com/article.cfm?id=eating-made-simple.

HANDOUT

STRATEGIES TO HELP CHILDREN ACHIEVE A HEALTHY WEIGHT

Obesity is caused by a number of factors that interact with each other in complex ways. These include (a) *environmental and policy factors,* such as the easy availability of low-cost, high-calorie foods and funding cuts to physical education programs; (b) *behavioral factors,* such as spending a lot of time watching television; and (c) *biological factors.* In the simplest terms, obesity results when we eat more calories than our bodies use repeatedly over time. Strategies to help children achieve and maintain a healthy weight focus on helping them eat healthy and be active.

Help Children Make Healthy Drink Choices

Liquid calories can add up quickly when drinking sugar-sweetened beverages and 100% fruit juice. Sugar-sweetened beverages that can contain large quantities of high fructose corn syrup include soda, fruit punch, lemonade, iced tea, flavored coffee drinks, and sports drinks.

- Parents and children should check the nutrition facts on the bottle's label to see how many calories a serving of their favorite drink contains.
- It is important to note that a drink bottle can contain multiple servings. To determine the total calories in a drink bottle, the calories for each serving need to be multiplied by the number of servings in the bottle. (For example, a drink may have 100 calories per 8-ounce serving; a 16-ounce bottle of this drink has 2 servings in it, so the entire bottle contains 200 calories).
- Some people may be surprised to find out that 100% fruit juice is relatively high in calories. The American Academy of Pediatrics recommends that toddlers and young children drink no more than 6 ounces of 100% fruit juice per day and that older children and adolescents limit their daily fruit juice intake to no more than 12 ounces. In addition to drinking water, low-fat milk, and limited amounts of juice, children can have fun making lower-calorie juice drinks by combining carbonated water (club soda or seltzer) with juice or by freezing juice in an ice cube tray and adding the frozen juice cubes to sparkling or plain tap water.

Help Children to Eat Plenty of Fruit, Vegetables, and Whole Grains

Encouraging children to eat diets that are high in fruit, vegetables, and whole grains can be challenging due to the higher costs of these foods, the relative unavailability of these foods in poorer communities, and the convenience of getting inexpensive meals at fast-food restaurants. The following ideas can help children develop healthy eating behaviors:

- Small changes, such as the type of snack foods bought, can be a good place to start to develop healthier eating behaviors. Fruit, vegetables, cheese, yogurt, and whole-grain crackers can be purchased in place of cakes, chips, doughnuts, candy, and cookies. Children can be involved in food shopping and food preparation.
- Parents are influential role models, so it is important that they make healthy eating choices around children.
- All foods can be enjoyed infrequently and in small quantities. Restricting foods only increases their value and makes children want them even more.
- Foods should not be used as a reward, as this only increases their value to a child.
- Many children are hesitant to eat foods that are new to them. Sometimes it can take 10 to 15 exposures to a new food before a young child likes it. Being persistent (but not pushy or forceful) in encouraging children to eat new foods by providing repeated exposures of small quantities can be helpful.

You can ask the child to take a "no thank you" bite of the new food if she or he does not want to eat it.

- Finally, parents should ask their child's health care provider how many calories he or she should consume each day for optimal growth and development. This number will depend on the child's age, gender, and level of physical activity.

Help Children Be Physically Active and Reduce Sedentary Activity or "Screen Time"

- The U.S. Department of Health and Human Services and the National Association for Sport and Physical Education recommend that school-age children and adolescents get at least 60 minutes of age-appropriate physical activity on all or most days of the week.
- Opportunities to engage in physical activity in recess and gym class should not be withheld as a punishment.
- Physical activities should be varied in nature and should occur multiple times per day, lasting at least 15 minutes per occasion. At school, physical education and structured recess programs are obvious places where children and adolescents can be active. Afterschool programs are another important place where children can be active. In addition, communities can organize Safe Routes to School programs to encourage walking and biking (see www.saferoutesinfo.org).
- Parents can advocate for expanded physical education programs at parent council meetings, if their child's school district does not provide physical education multiple times per week.
- Physical activity levels tend to decline during adolescence, so it is important to find ways to motivate teens to be active.
- Too much "screen time," including watching television, playing video games, or using the computer, has been linked to childhood overweight. The American Academy on Pediatrics recommends that children's "screen time" be limited to no more than 1 to 2 hours per day.

12

Low-Level Aggression in the Schools

Issues and Interventions

Rebecca Lakin Gullan, Julie Paquette MacEvoy, and Stephen S. Leff

Jenna is a 13-year-old, African-American girl attending school in an urban, impoverished neighborhood. Jenna's teacher describes her as "energetic" and "disorganized." She has been in the principal's office three times in the past month for being involved in loud and hostile arguments with other girls in her class. On one occasion, the verbal exchange escalated when Jenna shoved the other girl.

Jenna reports that she does not have any close friends and complains that other children pick on her and talk about her behind her back. Most recently, she said that when the class changed seats, the student she sat next to "moved way to the edge of his desk and gave [her] a dirty look." Jenna indicates that she wishes she had more friends and realizes that fighting is getting in the way with that. At the same time, Jenna feels that if she does not stand up for herself when other children are mean or aggressive toward her, things will escalate. Further, Jenna said that her mother and brothers encourage her to not back down, because it is a sign of weakness and she could get hurt badly.

Attempts by Jenna's teacher and other school staff (e.g., lunchroom aides) to monitor and intervene have been unsuccessful. Jenna's teacher reports that Jenna appears to provoke or escalate conflicts at times because "she thinks everyone is out to get her," and she "doesn't know when to stop."

INTRODUCTION

Low-level child aggression is a problem that continually challenges parents, psychologists, teachers, and other school staff. Issues related to child aggression are complex and require a comprehensive understanding of the characteristics, context, and consequences of behavior. With additional knowledge, educators can identify when the typical conflicts of childhood become problematic, how aggression manifests itself differently for boys and girls, the distinctive presentation of aggressive-victims, and the association between popularity and aggression.

BACKGROUND

Child aggression has been identified as a critical problem across continents and cultures. Although school shootings and other extreme acts of youth violence have received widespread attention, low-level aggression presents a daily challenge to those working in schools and related settings. Despite differences in the definition and measurement of aggression across studies and cultures, international research suggests that up to half of students are involved as the perpetrator or victim of aggression (Eslea et al., 2003). Further, the majority of students indicate having witnessed aggression between classmates (Bradshaw, Sawyer, & O'Brennan, 2007).

With regard to developmental differences, low-level aggression tends to be most prevalent in younger children, with the number of self-identified victims decreasing and the number of aggressors increasing with age (Solberg, Olweus, & Endresen, 2007). Girls and boys tend to be victims at the same rate, whereas boys are more frequently identified as aggressors or as aggressive-victims (Perren & Alsaker, 2006). Girls' involvement might be underestimated, however, due to an emphasis on direct or physical means of expressing aggression (e.g., hitting and pushing) as opposed to more social manifestations, such as starting rumors and being socially exclusive (Xu, Farver, Schwartz, & Chang, 2003).

What Is a Normal Level of Aggression?

Studies have found that school staff underreport the extent to which aggression occurs (as compared to child reports) and students feel that their schools do not provide sufficient intervention or prevention efforts. These findings might relate to the relatively high prevalence of aggression in unstructured settings where adults are less likely to be present (e.g., hallway, lunchroom, recess; Leff, Power, Costigan, & Manz, 2003). They could also reflect the belief that conflict between children is normative and adult intervention—particularly in the case of low-level aggression that does not present significant physical threat to a child—might impede social skill development. Yet engagement in even low-level aggression has been found to relate to negative outcomes, including a low sense of safety, poor expectations about the future, and the perpetration of more severe aggression (Boxer, Edwards-Leeper, Goldstein, Musher-Eizenman, & Dubow, 2003).

Conflict Versus Aggression. In considering when to intervene with low-level child aggression, it is critical to recognize the distinction between the common developmental experience of conflict and the choice to use aggression in response to conflict. Thus, although learning to cope effectively with interpersonal disagreements is an important developmental skill, aggression is only one potential reaction to conflict situations. Indeed, while the majority of children experience interpersonal disagreements, most respond with strategies other than aggression, such as persuasion or compromise. As such, helping children learn to cope with conflict involves the recognition that aggression is a response choice rather than an inevitable developmental experience.

Cultural Differences. Although child aggression has been identified as problematic across cultures, behavioral norms and social goals vary widely, thereby influencing the level of aggressive behavior considered acceptable and functional (Xu et al., 2003). For example, Chen and French (2008) indicated that self- and group-oriented cultures value behavioral control and social initiative to different degrees, resulting in different standards for social competence. Consequently, youth aggression in a collectivist culture (e.g., China) might be further outside the acceptable norm than it would be in an individualistic culture (e.g., the United States).

Classroom Differences. Students' aggressive behavior also varies related to their beliefs about what others in their class find acceptable. Children in classrooms where there is a higher level of aggressive behavior are more likely to behave aggressively themselves (Thomas, Bierman, & the Conduct Problems Prevention Research Group, 2006). Basic behavioral principles suggest that teacher attitudes and actions are also likely to influence the level of aggression within the classroom. For example, how a teacher responds when aggression occurs (e.g., a disapproving look, verbal reprimand, withdrawal of privileges, ignoring) can impact the likelihood of future aggressive acts.

Understanding the influence of factors outside the child (e.g., cultural or classroom context) has important implications for developing effective interventions. For example, addressing aggressive behavior in youth living in circumstances characterized by high levels of aggression—such as inner-city, impoverished neighborhoods—should take into account the context in which that behavior occurs.

Defining Nonphysical Aggression. A variety of terms have been used to describe the nonphysical ways in which students express anger and aggression toward one another, with two of the currently most popular labels being *relational aggression* and *social aggression*. Relational aggression includes behaviors that are used purposely to manipulate and damage someone's relationships, such as threatening to terminate a friendship, socially excluding a peer, and ignoring (Crick & Grotpeter, 1995). Galen and Underwood (1997) defined social aggression as any behaviors that function to harm the target's self-concept or social standing, including negative gossiping, friendship manipulation, and social exclusion. Unlike relational aggression, however, social aggression also includes nonverbal behaviors, such as nasty facial expressions and eye rolling, that have been shown to be hurtful to youth (Paquette & Underwood, 1999). Despite some definitional distinctions, these terms describe largely similar behaviors and are often used interchangeably.

Regardless of the term employed, girls have consistently been found to be more likely to aggress against peers by using negative gossiping, social exclusion, and friendship manipulation than by using physical forms of aggression (Galen & Underwood, 1997). Further, whereas girls engage in less physical aggression as they get older, they tend to display more indirectly aggressive behaviors over time. Importantly, several studies have shown that youth view socially and relationally aggressive acts to be extremely hurtful (Galen & Underwood). The frequency with which children are the targets of social aggression is negatively associated with feelings of self-competence (Paquette & Underwood, 1999), and the more often children are the victims of relational aggression, the greater their loneliness, depression, social anxiety, and social avoidance (Crick & Grotpeter, 1996).

Bullies, Victims, and Aggressive-Victims

Understanding low-level aggression necessitates discussion of the distinct yet overlapping literature on bullying. *Bullying* is defined as aggressive acts that are repeated over time and involve an imbalance of power. Although often used interchangeably with the term *aggression, bullying* emphasizes the power differential and repetitive nature of the aggressive acts. One critical group of youth identified in the bullying literature is those who are both aggressors and victims, also known as bully-victims or provocative-victims.

Bully-Victims. In general, 7% to 15% of youth identify themselves as bullies, 10% as victims, and 2% to 15% as bully-victims (Pellegrini, Bartini, & Brooks, 1999). Youth who at times are the perpetrators of peer aggression but at other times are the victims are a critical subgroup who present with an especially challenging constellation of behaviors and are at high risk for problematic short- and long-term outcomes.

Bully-victims are characterized by traits of both victims and aggressors. Similar to aggressors, bully-victims exhibit externalizing behaviors (i.e., problem behaviors directed toward others, usually aggressively; Kokkinos & Panayiotou, 2004). Consistent with victims, on the other hand, bully-victims are less social than other children and have fewer friends, even as early as kindergarten (Perren & Alsaker, 2006). Thus, while bullies do not appear to have significant social disadvantages (e.g., smaller friendship networks) or low self-esteem and victims do not exhibit externalizing problems, children who are both bullies and victims demonstrate deficits across both domains. As such, bully-victims have been found to have higher distress levels and more difficulty regulating their emotions than children who are just bullies or just victims and to experience more social rejection (Schwartz, 2000). Bully-victims experience victimization across other life domains as well (e.g., crime, maltreatment, and sexual victimization). Although increased victimization rates also occur for children who are bullies or victims only, the rates for bully-victims are higher.

Aggression and Social Status: The Role of Perceived Popularity

Although aggression is typically linked with low popularity and poor outcomes, such as loneliness, depression, school dropout, and delinquency (Crick & Grotpeter, 1995), there appears to be a subset of youth who are both aggressive and of high social status. This highlights the distinction between defining *popularity* as being liked by peers (sociometric popularity) versus being viewed by peers as being cool or popular (perceived popularity). Interestingly, sociometrically popular youth (those who are well liked) are not always the same as those who are perceived to be popular but are not necessarily well liked (Parkhurst & Hopmeyer, 1998). In fact, only one third of youth who are sociometrically popular (peers say they like them) are also perceived as popular (peers say they are popular; Cillessen & Rose, 2005).

Youth who are aggressive but perceived to be popular appear to be better adjusted than youth who are aggressive and rejected by their peers (Cillessen & Rose, 2005). Boys who are aggressive but perceived to be popular do not show elevated levels of internalizing symptoms (i.e., inwardly directed emotional issues, such as anxiety and depression). In addition, youth who are highly relationally aggressive but are seen as popular have better quality friendships than youth who are relationally aggressive and disliked by their peers. Some scholars have suggested that although perceived-popular youth may not be at risk for maladjustment in the short term, they may have poor long-term outcomes. Indeed, perceived popularity has been shown to predict engagement in risky behaviors, such as alcohol use and sexual activity, in adolescence, suggesting that despite their high status in the peer group, perceived popular youth who are aggressive may be in need of intervention (Mayeux, Sandstrom, & Cillessen, 2008). Effective interventions for aggressive youth who are perceived as popular, however, might differ from those interventions intended for aggressive children who are rejected by their peers.

IMPLICATIONS FOR EDUCATORS

Successful intervention for low-level aggression and bullying requires evaluating and targeting each of the key factors discussed above. As such, those working with children should consider the characteristics of the child; the context in which the behavior occurs; and the form, function, and consequences of the aggressive behavior.

Evaluation at the Child Level

The research on youth aggression clearly indicates that all youth who are involved in aggressive or bullying exchanges are not the same.

1. School personnel must identify the role of the child in the aggressive exchanges (e.g., aggressor, victim, or aggressive-victim), because this role directly relates to child outcomes and effective interventions.

2. The types of aggression the youth engages in should be considered with sensitivity to the different forms of aggression (i.e., relational, physical, or verbal).

3. The venue in which aggressive exchanges take place (e.g., classroom, playground, or over the Internet or cell phone) must also be considered.

4. The social status (e.g., popular versus rejected) of aggressive children should be taken into consideration.

Knowledge of each of these four factors will help to tailor an intervention that will be maximally effective for each individual child. For example, intervention for a popular girl who starts rumors about her peers will be different than helping a rejected boy who hits and kicks his classmates on the playground.

Evaluating Context

An important consideration in evaluating aggressive behavior is the context in which the behavior occurs. Norms at the ethnic/cultural, neighborhood, and classroom level have a strong influence on children's attitudes toward aggression, which subsequently influence their behavior (Roberto, Meyer, Boster, & Roberto, 2003). As such, evaluation of cultural and classroom norms can be informative as to types or levels of aggressive behavior are considered acceptable within the child's social environment. For example, if a child is 1 of 20 aggressors in a classroom of 25 students, a classwide intervention system might be more effective than if that child is the only identified aggressor.

Another consideration when evaluating youth involved in peer aggression or bullying is the need to screen for problems outside of the social realm. Youth who are involved in bullying and aggression—and particularly those who are both bullies and victims—have been found to have a multitude of problems across other realms, including academic, behavioral, and psychological functioning. It follows that effective interventions must also address potential issues beyond aggression.

Matching Intervention to Child and Contextual Characteristics

A number of aggression and bullying interventions take place across schools every day. Few, however, meet the criteria for being empirically validated interventions, and even fewer are tailored to the specific needs of the child and the context (Leff et al., 2003). Nonetheless, practitioners who carefully evaluate key factors related to the child and his or her context will subsequently be able to identify specific intervention goals. These goals can then be matched with empirically supported or promising interventions expected to produce maximal success.

Prevention. In preventing aggressive behavior, it is critical that adults identify opportunities where children can be taught appropriate and effective skills to resolve conflicts. Parental intervention in sibling conflict decreased the conflict and led to greater sophistication in child behavior (Chen & French, 2008). Informal intervention can promote social development through modeling problem solving and self-control. Adult engagement also provides opportunity for teaching incremental skills that expand the child's social problem-solving capacity. More formal aggression prevention programs are also a mechanism for students to learn and practice pro-social problem solving, anger management, and conflict resolution skills.

Intervening With Victims. Research on victims of aggression suggests that they have fewer friends and lower self-esteem and are more isolated and lonely than their peers (Perren & Alsaker, 2006). In addition, they tend to have deficits in social problem solving (Cassidy & Taylor, 2005). As such, it is critically important that victims of bullying be provided with social support and connection with others, as well as opportunities to develop social problem-solving skills so they can maintain relationships over time. Such friendships are likely to be protective not only in terms of future mental health but also in coping with bullying situations when they occur (Perren & Alsaker).

Intervening With Aggressors. Youth who are primarily aggressors engage in proactive (unprovoked) acts against other children in pursuit of two primary goals: domination and social approval. Aggressors have also been identified as having deficits in the response choice and enactment steps of Crick and Dodge's (1994) social information processing (SIP) model, wherein they are less able than other children to generate pro-social responses to social problems, they view aggression and its outcomes more positively, and they feel greater efficacy for engaging in aggressive acts. Aggressive youth might also see ambiguous acts as having hostile intent (Dodge, 1980). Thus, interventions for children who are primarily aggressors should target the following five factors outlined by Crick and Dodge (1996):

1. Change social norms/acceptability.

2. Control contingencies for aggressive behavior.

3. Identify more appropriate social goals.

4. Teach alternatives to aggressive behaviors.

5. Encourage youth to consider nonhostile explanations for the actions of others.

For example, teachers might establish clear rules around aggressive behavior in the classroom. Other children should also be encouraged to reject aggression and bullying behavior and work together to meet common goals. Helping aggressive children to channel their desire for dominance into pro-social activities (e.g., leadership) might also be effective, particularly for aggressive children who are perceived as popular by their peers. Finally, aggressive youth should be taught that there are more effective and less harmful ways to respond to social problems and be encouraged and reinforced for implementing pro-social solutions.

Intervening With Bully-Victims. As described above, youth who are both aggressors and victims of aggression appear to be a distinct subgroup of children with difficulties that span those experienced by both bullies and victims alike. It follows that any suggested interventions for bully-victims coincide with those prescribed for victims (e.g., building social networks, teaching social problem-solving skills) as well as bullies (e.g., increasing prosocial response choice and enactment). In particular, bully-victims, who tend to be emotionally dysregulated and reactive, should be taught how to calm themselves and consider situations carefully before responding. Further, the related academic and behavioral deficits of bully-victims require that attention be paid to functioning outside of the social realm, including attending to problems in the home environment and addressing learning difficulties. Finally, bully-victims appear to have particular deficits in the step of the SIP model wherein they interpret social cues. Thus, bully-victims are more likely to attribute hostile intent to others' behavior or situations. For example, a child with a hostile attribution bias who is bumped in the hallway is more likely to assume the other child did it on purpose and to react accordingly (Crick & Dodge, 1996). Consequently, interventions with bully-victims should focus on helping them consider alternate explanations for provocative situations so as to halt the impulsive aggression response characteristic of these children.

Changing Social Norms. Underlying efforts to decrease problems with aggression and bullying for all children is the need to address social and cultural norms. On the classroom or school level, this involves increased efforts to socialize children in the direction of cooperative behavior and decrease acceptance of aggression (Chen & French, 2008). One way to do this is to address adult attitudes and beliefs about aggression, such as how normal is it or when (if ever) it is justified (Bradshaw et al., 2007). Given the influence that teachers have over classroom norms, either explicitly (e.g., verbal direction, class rules) or implicitly (e.g., disapproving looks, classroom organization), teachers' attitudes about aggression are likely to influence greatly subsequent child beliefs and behaviors (Henry, 2001).

EDUCATIONAL STRATEGIES

- Effective intervention strategies depend on individual child factors; that is, whether the child is the aggressor, victim, or aggressive-victim and whether the child engages in verbal, physical, or indirect aggression.
- Context must also be considered. For example, what are the cultural and classroom norms for different types of aggressive behavior?
- Academic, behavioral, and psychological functioning should be considered when working with youth who have social problems.
- Adult modeling and teaching of problem-solving skills can help to prevent or mitigate aggression.

DISCUSSION QUESTIONS

1. If you were working with a child who engaged in low-level aggression but appeared to be well adjusted and popular with peers, would you be less likely to intervene than you would with a child who engages in low-level aggression but is exhibiting adjustment problems and has few friends? Why or why not? In which case is an intervention more urgent or necessary?

2. Would you be less likely to intervene with a popular child who engages in relational aggression than with a popular child who engages in low-level physical or verbal aggression?

3. Some people believe that we have gone too far in intervening in bullying/aggressive exchanges between youth and that we are standing in the way of children learning how to handle conflict on their own. Do you agree or disagree with this and why? At what point do you feel intervention is necessary?

4. If controlling contingencies (e.g., punishing aggressive behavior, reinforcing pro-social behavior) for children who are bullies effectively eliminates aggression, do you feel this is sufficient? Or should interventionists attempt to change the bullies' attitudes or beliefs as well?

RESEARCH SUMMARY

- Low-level aggression is prevalent in our schools.
- Expected or typical levels of aggression depend on cultural and classroom context.
- Girls more often engage in nonphysical forms of aggression, also known as indirect, relational, or social aggression.
- Children might be bullies, victims, or bully-victims, each of which has different outcomes.
- Youth who are primarily aggressors engage in proactive (unprovoked) acts against other children in pursuit of two primary goals: domination and social approval.
- Youth who are aggressive but perceived to be popular are better adjusted than youth who are aggressive and rejected by their peers.
- Children who are aggressive but also perceived as popular or "cool" tend to have better outcomes than those rated as aggressive and rejected.

RESOURCES

Sheras, P. (2002). *Your child: Bully or victim? Understanding and ending schoolyard tyranny.* New York: Skylight.

The following Web site from the U.S. Health Resources and Services Administration presents resources for children to use to address bullying, as well as bibliographies and links to additional resources:

Stop Bullying Now!: www.stopbullyingnow.hrsa.gov

HANDOUT

HELPING CHILDREN WITH AGGRESSION

Children who are involved in aggressive exchanges do so in a number of different ways and for many different reasons. Consequently, successful intervention involves a two-step process. First, we must identify the form and function of the behavior, the social status of the child, and the context in which the aggressive behavior occurs. Second, information on form, function, status, and context must be matched to interventions that address the difficulties specific to that child.

STEP 1: What Is Happening?

1. What type of aggression is the child involved in: physical, verbal, indirect/social/relational (such as leaving others out, spreading rumors), or a combination?

2. Is the child an aggressor, a victim, or both an aggressor and a victim?

3. Is the child considered popular by peers?

4. In what context does the behavior take place?
   a. Do others think it is okay or normal to be aggressive?
   b. Do others engage in aggressive behavior?
   c. How do adults respond (or not respond) to aggression?

5. What is the broader context? For example, what are neighborhood levels of violence, or what is considered acceptable or normal for the child's cultural group?

STEP 2: Intervention Based on Evaluation

1. *Social/Relational Aggression.* If child is engaging in an indirect form of aggression, (1) teach the child that behaviors such as threatening to withdraw friendship and eye rolling are also forms of aggression and (2) emphasize that it is possible to be hurtful without hitting or yelling at someone.

2. *Aggressor.* If child is the aggressor (1) change what is considered acceptable behavior (e.g., have rules that emphasize cooperation); (2) reward helpful, friendly behavior and punish aggression; (3) identify more appropriate social goals (e.g., leadership): (4) teach alternatives to aggressive behaviors (e.g., compromise, problem solving); and (5) encourage consideration of nonhostile explanations for the actions of others (e.g., if someone bumps into you in the hallway, assume it was an accident). If the child is considered popular by peers, provide opportunities for positive leadership.

3. *Victim.* If the child is the victim, (1) teach assertiveness skills, (2) teach social skills (e.g., how to enter a game or activity) and problem solving, and (3) build social support.

4. *Aggressive-Victim.* If the child is an aggressor and a victim, (1) provide assertiveness and social skills training, (2) build social support, (3) encourage thinking of alternatives to hostile explanations for others' behavior, (4) teach problem solving, and (5) address any additional problems, such as academic or emotional difficulties.

5. *Aggressive Context.* If many children are exhibiting aggression in a specific place or time, such as a classroom, (1) change classroom norms and expectations, (2) remove reinforcement (the payoff), and (3) institute consequences for aggression.

13

Accident Prevention

MaryBeth Bailar-Heath and Sarah Valley-Gray

Anthony is a 10-year-old male in a single-parent home comprising of his mother and three siblings. He and his two younger brothers and one younger sister attend public school in a low-income neighborhood. Anthony's mother drives the children to school each morning on her way to work. Anthony rides in the front seat of the family car. His mother argues with him each day to wear his seatbelt, but he says it is uncomfortable and refuses to wear it. They are usually running late, so his mother tends to give in to prevent an argument.

At school, Anthony's favorite time of the day is recess. He plays football and basketball with the other boys. Anthony prefers to play with the older boys in his neighborhood as opposed to children his own age. In fact, some of his recess playmates are 13 years old. Anthony's mother is still at work when school is dismissed, so Anthony is responsible for walking his younger siblings home from school, nearly a mile away. Anthony gets bored with the same route, so he likes to take different paths. When the children arrive home, Anthony prepares a snack for his siblings. Then he usually plays outdoors with the neighborhood children. Anthony's mother returns from work by dinnertime.

Anthony's daily routine is not that different from that of many other students at his elementary school. A teacher at the school saw the need for developing an accident prevention program to target many of the risk factors she noticed in the students' daily routines, environments, and family life. First, a motor vehicle safety program was implemented that included informational sessions for parents and checkpoints on the school property where children were dropped off and picked up (to check for proper use of safety seats and backseat riding). Recess times were restructured so that students were on the playground only with relatively same-age peers. Finally, the teacher spearheaded an afterschool program with community volunteers to ensure that children had appropriate supervision until they were picked up by their parents or guardians after work.

INTRODUCTION

Accidental injury is the leading cause of death among children 5 to 19 years of age in the United States. Although accidental injuries are more prevalent than violence-related injuries and result in more childhood deaths than homicide and suicide combined, minimal attention is provided to the prevention of such accidents in our schools, communities, and neighborhoods.

Of all the causes of unintentional injuries, motor vehicle accidents are the most frequent cause of mortality in the school-age population, followed by pedestrian and bicycling accidents. Prevention of sports- and recreation-related injuries is also important, as these are the most frequently occurring injuries on school property. Traumatic brain injury and spinal cord injury are common, and chronic outcomes of many accidents have significant effects on development, academics, and behavior.

BACKGROUND

Motor Vehicle Safety

The Centers for Disease Control and Prevention (CDC) reports that motor vehicle accidents are the leading cause of death from injuries among children and adolescents between the ages of 5 and 19 years in the United States. In fact, 70% of deaths of children and teens are caused by motor vehicle crashes. Additionally, approximately 1.5 million children and adolescents are seen in hospital emergency departments annually due to injuries from motor vehicle crashes (CDC, 2001). The research surrounding motor vehicle safety is clear. The proper use of child safety seats, booster seats, and seat belts prevents and reduces injuries to children in motor vehicle accidents (Durbin, Elliot, & Winston, 2003). Problems arise when these safety devices are not used properly or at all (Staunton et al., 2005).

A systematic review of the literature investigating motor vehicle accident prevention programs targeted at increasing child safety seat use yields several important recommendations (Zaza et al., 2005). First, the implementation of child safety seat laws is recommended, given the strong evidence for its effectiveness. Child safety seat laws can reduce the total number of injuries to children by approximately 35% and increase safety seat use by 13% (Zaza et al.). Second, distribution of and education programs about child safety seats are recommended. These programs may help to increase rates of correct child safety seat use by approximately 23%. However, programs that lend or distribute seats must use only new products, as the safety of refurbished ones cannot be guaranteed (Zaza et al.).

Pedestrian Safety

In addition to motor vehicle passenger injury, pedestrian injury can be another result of traffic-related accidents. Approximately 630 child pedestrian deaths and 39,000 nonfatal child pedestrian injuries occur annually, suggesting the importance of teaching children pedestrian safety skills (Safe Kids Worldwide, 2007).

Children under the age of 10 should not be allowed to cross the street without adult supervision (NSKC, 2005). Therefore, the most important pedestrian injury prevention strategy before the age of 10 is adequate supervision by an adult when children are playing, walking, or engaging in other activities near streets. Even when preparing to cross the street with an adult, children should be instructed to look left, right, and left again before crossing and to stay alert for traffic while crossing. Additionally, play in unfenced yards, driveways, and streets should be prohibited. Finally, when an adult is walking with a young child, pedestrian skills such as safe street-crossing behavior should always be modeled appropriately.

When children reach the age of 10, they are usually developmentally prepared to begin learning how to cross streets safely. Independently, children should be taught to look left, right, and left again before crossing any streets, and to continue watching for traffic while crossing the street. They should only cross the street at corners, using stop signs, street lights, or crosswalks. Traffic signs and signals must also be understood. A child should be able to demonstrate knowledge and practice of all of these skills before he or she is allowed to cross streets independently (NSKC, 2005).

In an interesting and somewhat paradoxical study, Jacobsen (2003) compared the rate of walking and bicycling that occurred in given areas to the rate of pedestrian injuries. The incidence of a person who is walking or cycling being struck by a motorist varied inversely with the amount of walking/cycling that took place in that area. This pattern was consistent across communities of varying size, whether metropolitan or rural, and across time periods. Jacobsen posited that motorists adjust their behaviors in the presence of greater numbers of people walking and bicycling. Therefore, policies that increase the number of people walking and cycling (e.g., creating walking and biking paths) appear to be an effective method for improving the safety of pedestrians and cyclists.

Bicycle Safety

Between the years of 2001 and 2003, 357,590 children and teenagers were treated in emergency departments for bicycle injuries in the United States (Conn, Annest, Bossarte, & Gilchrist, 2006). Approximately 250 children and adolescents between the age of 5 and 19 are killed annually as a result of bicycle-related accidents. Children ages 10 to 14 years are responsible for 64% to 86% of bicycle-related fatalities and severe head injuries (CDC, 2001). The research is clear; helmet use reduces the risk of head injury among cyclists by 70% to 88% (Klassen, MacKay, Moher, Walker, & Jones, 2000). One extensive review of the literature identified the use of helmets when bicycling as one of the single best strategies to prevent mild head injury (Cassidy et al., 2004).

Given the clear evidence for the effectiveness of bicycle helmets in reducing injury and death, many prevention programs have targeted increasing their use among child and adolescent bicyclers. The most successful programs use multiple strategies targeted at different audiences to address the lack of awareness regarding the risks of bicycling and the effectiveness of helmets (Klassen et al., 2000). For example, educational interventions coupled with economic incentives, as well as educational interventions combined with legislation, are sound approaches. Strategies that use education as the sole intervention are not very effective. In contrast, programs that incorporate legislation requiring helmet use (e.g., ticketing when a helmet is not worn) result in the greatest increase in the behavior. Additionally, successful programs address negative peer pressure that may discourage other children from wearing helmets. It is also important to reduce financial barriers to purchasing a helmet, as children in low-income communities are often at higher risk of unintentional injury. Peer pressure has a significant influence on helmet usage, regardless of socioeconomic status. Children are more likely to wear a helmet if their friends or supervising adults wear one as well (Klassen et al.).

Many programs aim to prevent serious and fatal bicycle injuries in children by focusing not just on helmet usage but also on bicycle safety skills in general. An extensive review of such educational programs reported that the most comprehensive programs include traffic rules, safety guidelines, on-bike training, and helmet education in their curricula (Rivara & Metrik, 1998).

Sports, Recreation, and Swimming Safety

Sports and Recreation Safety. Play and recreational activities vary significantly among preschoolers, elementary schoolchildren, and adolescents. Therefore, risk factors and the most appropriate injury prevention strategies for each age group vary as well. For children up to 5 years of age, adequate supervision during play is the most important accident prevention strategy. Young children's curiosity and impulsivity make supervision by a responsible adult imperative, and children should never play unsupervised.

Children ages 5 to 9 years are at the greatest risk for sports and recreational injuries in the following areas: playground, bicycling, trampoline, scooter, and baseball/softball (Conn et al., 2006). Because children in this age range participate in much of their recreational activity on a playground, maintaining a safe play environment is important. Developing and enforcing appropriate safety rules, as well as ensuring adequate adult supervision, are key strategies to preventing accidental injury, regardless of the activity.

For children between 10 and 17 years of age, sports become the biggest area of recreational injury. More specifically, the most frequently occurring recreational injuries in this age group occur during basketball, football, baseball/softball, and soccer (Conn et al., 2006). The CDC (2001) reported that approximately 1 million serious sports-related injuries occur annually to children and adolescents between the ages of 10 and 17 years. Furthermore, sports cause more than half of all nonfatal injuries on school property, and approximately 300,000 mild to moderate traumatic brain injuries are classified as sports related each year. The highest rate of sports- and recreation-related traumatic brain injury emergency department visits for both males and females occurs among children between the ages of 10 and 14 years (CDC, 2007b).

The importance of protective equipment for children in sports cannot be overstated. A lack of awareness regarding potential injury, inappropriate or unavailable equipment, and lack of financial resources to purchase equipment are some of the barriers to injury prevention.

Additionally, parents should be encouraged to implement the same safety measures that they employ in games during practices, as most sports-related injuries occur during practices rather than games (NSKC, 2004).

Swimming Safety. Water recreation is another activity where accidents can result in injury and fatality. In fact, following traffic-related accidents, drowning is the second leading cause of unintentional injury-related death among children ages 1 to 14 years of age (CDC, 2001). Just as in sports and other play activities, the areas that pose the most danger vary according to a child's development.

In addition to supervision by a trained lifeguard, swimming lessons may help prevent drowning in children and adolescents. It is recommended that children be taught to swim no earlier than age 5 years, as children age 4 years and younger typically are not developmentally prepared to understand formal swimming instruction (Mayo Clinic, 2007). Studies have demonstrated that swimming lessons improve one's ability to dive, swim underwater, breathe correctly, and tread water (HIPRC, 2001).

Traumatic Brain Injury and Spinal Cord Injury

Children who sustain and survive accidents as discussed in this chapter could experience lifelong consequences in the form of a traumatic brain injury (TBI) or spinal cord injury (SCI). In fact, the two age groups at highest risk for TBI are children from birth to 4 years of age and adolescents from 15 to 19 years of age. The CDC estimates that at least 475,000 children ages birth to 14 years sustain a TBI annually in the United States. These brain injuries in children account for 37,000 hospitalizations and 435,000 emergency department visits annually. Approximately 2,700 of these children do not survive (Langlois, Rutland-Brown, & Thomas, 2004).

Children who survive a brain injury can experience a wide range of functional changes impacting thinking and intelligence, motor skills, sensation, language, and emotion. Given that children are in the midst of rapid developmental changes in all domains of functioning, including physical, cognitive, and behavioral, the neurological impairments resulting from a TBI can hinder future learning and cognitive development. In fact, recent research suggests that while children may appear to demonstrate less damage than adults early in recovery, deficits often emerge later as the child matures (Cronin, 2001).

Although SCI is less prevalent in childhood than TBI, this type of injury does occur and can be serious. SCI most often results from motor vehicle accidents. Additionally, sports and recreation activities cause an estimated 18% of SCI cases (NCIPC, 2006). Although some SCI cases result in almost complete recovery, others result in total paralysis. Individuals who survive SCI will most likely have medical complications such as chronic pain and bladder and bowel dysfunction along with an increased susceptibility to respiratory and heart problems (CDC, 2007b). Pressure sores, urinary tract infections, and scoliosis also commonly occur. Rehabilitation programs are usually needed for individuals who survive an SCI to address physical issues as well as social and emotional functioning (NCIPC).

IMPLICATIONS FOR EDUCATORS

Given the incidence and prevalence of accidental injuries among children and adolescents, it is important that educators understand the significance of accident prevention and, in particular, evidence-based strategies that can be implemented with their students.

Although school personnel can and should educate their students about accident prevention, the literature shows that education alone does not seem to be effective in decreasing accidental injuries or in increasing the use of appropriate safety measures. Broad-based, community interventions with multiple layers of involvement appear most effective. Schools have a responsibility to prevent injuries on school property and to teach students pertinent skills to promote safety (CDC, 2001). However, schools cannot and should not be expected to tackle the huge issue of childhood and adolescent accident prevention alone (CDC, 2007a). Instead, teachers and school staff should partner with the community.

The CDC (2007a) promotes the use of a coordinated school health program. Such a program includes eight components: health education, physical education, health services, nutrition services, psychological and counseling services, a healthy school environment, health promotion for school staff, and involvement of families and the community. A coordinated school health program promotes collaboration of school personnel, students, families, community organizations, agencies, and businesses in the development, implementation, and evaluation of childhood accident prevention efforts (CDC, 2001).

EDUCATIONAL STRATEGIES

- Educate teachers, staff, and parents about the importance of accident prevention, as it is the leading cause of death of children and adolescents from 5 to 19 years of age.
- Have safety lessons for students take place over the entire school year as opposed to one short period of the year. Merge accident prevention into already existing classroom lessons. For example, in a physics lesson, a teacher can explore the energy exchanges that take place in motor vehicle or bicycle crashes and how seat belts and helmets absorb energy. In art class, students may bring in their bike helmets to decorate with paint and stickers.
- Create family homework assignments to accompany the in-class safety curricula.
- Use active learning strategies, interactive teaching methods, and positive classroom management to encourage student participation in learning about unintentional injury. For example, incorporate supervised practice using safety devices and skills, discussion, cooperative learning, rehearsal, positive reinforcement, and role-playing.
- Remember to tailor educational programs to the culture and community in which your school is located. These programs also can help students understand social influences on health and safety-related behaviors and how to resist cultural, media, and peer pressure to make unsafe choices.

- Create a coordinated school health program to develop, implement, and evaluate accident prevention efforts. This program should comprise a team of teachers, school staff and administrators, students and their families, and community members and organizations.

DISCUSSION QUESTIONS

1. There is limited published research pertaining to effective accident prevention interventions for children. Why might this be? What about this research may make it difficult to carry out? What are some possible strategies to address these difficulties?

2. What are some ways to convey to parents the importance of accident prevention for their children?

3. In what ways can the community contribute to accident prevention for children? How can schools motivate the community to become involved in this effort?

4. What specific strategies could make education about accident prevention more hands-on and appealing to children and their parents?

5. A child is much more likely to be injured or killed from an accident than as a result of violence. However, violence in schools continues to receive significantly more attention from the media and the community and may even motivate more prevention efforts than accidental injury. Why might this be? How might the importance of accident prevention be communicated to and given more attention by schools, families of children, and the general public?

RESEARCH SUMMARY

- Accidental injury is the leading cause of death among children and adolescents from 5 to 19 years of age in the United States. These injuries are more prevalent than violence-related injuries, and they result in more child and adolescent deaths than homicide and suicide combined.
- Motor vehicle accidents are the most prevalent type of accidental injury to children and adolescents and result in 70% of the deaths in this population. The proper use of child safety seats, booster seats, and seat belts prevents and reduces injuries and deaths of children and adolescents in motor vehicle accidents.
- Pedestrian safety skills should be tailored and taught to children appropriately for their developmental level. Strategies include providing adequate supervision, conducting street-crossing training, and having the child demonstrate the ability to cross a street safely before being allowed to do so alone.
- Bicycle injuries and fatalities are dramatically reduced and prevented by a single prevention strategy, appropriate helmet use. In fact, helmet use reduces the risk of head injury by up to 88%.

- Sports and recreation safety strategies should be implemented with children and adolescents appropriately for their developmental level. Strategies include adequate supervision, a safe play environment, and the use of protective gear or equipment.

RESOURCES

Frumkin, H., Geller, R. J., & Rubin, I. L. (Eds.). (2006). *Safe and healthy school environments*. New York: Oxford Press.

Mares, B. (2004). *Child safety 101*. Bloomington, IN: Unlimited.

Marotz, L. R. (2008). *Health, safety, and nutrition for the young child* (7th ed.). Cliffton Park, NY: Cengage Delmar Learning.

Robertson, C. (2006). *Safety, nutrition and health in early education* (3rd ed.). Albany, NY: Thomas Delmar Learning.

Silverstein, A., Silverstein, V. B., & Nunn, L. S. (2000). *Staying safe*. New York: Grolier.

H A N D O U T

TIPS FOR PREVENTING ACCIDENTAL INJURY OF CHILDREN AND ADOLESCENTS

Accidental injury is the leading cause of death among children from 5 to 19 years of age in the United States. The two age groups at highest risk for traumatic brain injury as a result of an accident are children from birth to 4 years and 15- to 19-year-olds. Motor vehicle, pedestrian, and bicycle accidents are commonly occurring events that cause injuries and fatalities among children. However, many of these injuries can be prevented by taking simple precautions. Adequately supervising children and modeling safety behaviors are essential. Parents and educators can work with schools and communities to develop and implement quality accident prevention programs.

Child Passenger Safety

- All children ages 12 and under should ride in the back seat of the car.
- Children who weigh 40 to 80 pounds should be seated in a booster seat and restrained with lap and shoulder belts every time they are traveling in a car.
- Typically, children weighing over 80 pounds and at least 8 years of age can fit correctly in lap/shoulder belts. The lap belt should fit across the child's hips (not the stomach) when the child is sitting against the vehicle seat. The shoulder belt should cross the center of the shoulder. Do not let children put shoulder belts under their arms or behind their backs, as this could result in serious injury.
- Always wear your seat belt for your own safety and to model this behavior for the child.

Bicycle Safety

- Children should not be taught to ride a bicycle (without training wheels) until 5 years of age.
- Ensure that children always wear helmets. Helmet use reduces the risk of head injury in the event of an accident by nearly 90%. You should wear a helmet too, not only for your own safety but as a model for the child.
- Allow the child to decorate his or her helmet with paint and stickers to make wearing it more fun.
- Make sure that the child's helmet fits properly. The helmet should sit on top of the child's head in a level position, cover his or her forehead, and not rock forward and backward or from side to side. The straps should be fastened. Bring the child to the store to try on a helmet before purchasing one.
- Teach children to stop at all stop signs, look both ways, and know when it is safe to cross a street. Bicycle with the child to show where riding is allowed. Children need to know to ride with traffic flow as far to the right as possible and how to gesture properly and make left-hand turns.
- Children younger than 10 years of age should ride on sidewalks instead of the street.
- Regularly check the child's bike to make sure the wheels, seat, and handlebars are all tight; the brakes are working appropriately; and the chain is tight.

Pedestrian Safety

Children should be taught the following rules:

- Do not cross the street alone if you are younger than 10 years of age.
- Stop at the curb before crossing the street.
- Walk—don't run—across the street.
- Cross at corners, using traffic signals and crosswalks.
- Look left, right, and left again before crossing. Be sure to remain alert when crossing.
- Walk facing traffic.
- Make sure drivers see you before crossing in front of them.

- Do not play in driveways, streets, parking lots, or unfenced yards by the street.
- Wear white clothing or reflectors when walking at night.

Sports and Recreation

- Check playgrounds where children play. Look for age-appropriate equipment and hazards such as rusted or broken equipment and dangerous surfaces. Report any hazards to the school or municipality.
- Teach children the importance of appropriate playground behavior: no pushing, shoving, or crowding.
- Remove hoods and neck drawstrings from children's outerwear to avoid strangulation hazards on playgrounds.
- Before beginning a sport, a child should have a general physical exam.
- Make sure that children are supervised at all times during sports games and practices.
- Ensure that when engaging in sports, children wear appropriately fitting safety gear and equipment.

Water Safety

Children should learn to swim (at age 5 or older) through the local department of parks and recreation or a Red Cross chapter. They should be taught the following rules:

- Wear U.S. Coast Guard-approved life jackets. (Inflatable inner tubes or "water rings" should not be used as safety devices.)
- Always swim with a buddy.
- Never go near a pool drain with or without a cover. Pin up long hair when in the water.
- Never run, push, or jump on others around water.
- Swim only within designated safe areas of rivers, lakes, and oceans and only where lifeguards are present.
- Never dive into a river, lake, or ocean.

Glossary

Chapter 2

Collaboration—A process by which two or more people or groups work together toward a common goal. For example, collaboration may occur between a child's parents and teachers to create a behavioral treatment plan in the home and classroom.

Consultation—A process by which a person or group seeks the expertise of a professional

Diagnostic and Statistical Manual of Mental Disorders, **text revision** **(DSM-IV-TR)**—A reference book for psychologists and other mental health professionals published by the American Psychiatric Association that describes the diagnostic criteria for mental disorders

Health Insurance Portability and Accountability Act of 1996 (HIPAA)— A complex federal law with important protections for the confidentiality and communication of medical records between professionals and systems

Individuals with Disabilities Education Act (IDEA)—A federal law in the United States that governs how states and public agencies provide services, such as early intervention and special education, to children with disabilities

International Classification of Disease (ICD-10)—A system used by physicians and other medical professionals that provides codes to classify disease

Medical-Educational Liaison—Ensures effective communication between two parties, such as between educators and medical professionals. Teachers who work in hospital-based classrooms, school nurses, school psychologists, and other professionals who have experience in both medical and educational environments can act as liaisons.

Chapter 3

Acoustic Reflex Measurement—A test of the middle ear, known as an acoustic immittance measure. It is used to detect hearing loss and to determine other diagnostic information about the middle ear. It can be conducted with young children who otherwise could not voluntarily participate in a hearing screening.

Allergic Rhinitis—Occurs when dust, dander, or plant pollens cause a reaction in the nose that triggers the release of histamines. This causes swelling and fluid production in the nose, sinuses, and eyes in people who are allergic to such substances.

Grapheme—Basic unit of written language, such as the letter *A*

Hearing Tone Tests (also known as pure-tone audiometry)—Used to evaluate the faintest tones a person can hear at selected pitches (frequencies) from low to high. During hearing tone tests, earphones are worn, and sound travels through the air in the ear canal to stimulate the eardrum and then the auditory nerve.

Myringotomy—A surgery performed to alleviate chronic ear infections. The surgery involves placing pressure equalization tubes into the middle ear. The tubes allow air to enter the middle ear space, which allows the lining of the middle ear to heal, preventing future infections. The tubes stay in place for 6 to 12 months and eventually fall out on their own.

Phoneme—Basic unit of written language that has meaning, such as the sound of a letter

Speech Audiometry—Used to determine speech reception threshold and to test word recognition.

Speech Reception Threshold—Testing used to determine the faintest level of sound (in decibels) at which a person can hear and correctly repeat common two-syllable words, such as *softball*

Tympanometry—A test of the middle ear, known as an acoustic immittance measure. It is used to detect fluid in the middle ear, damage of the ear drum, and/or wax blocking the ear canal.

Word Recognition Test—Determines how well a person can differentiate words at a comfortable loudness level.

Chapter 4

Antigen—A substance that promotes the generation of antibodies and promotes an immune response

Hemophilus Influenza B (Hib)—A bacterial infection that can result in meningitis and pneumonia. It most often affects infants and children.

Chapter 5

Anterior Fontanels—The soft spot on the top front of a baby's head where the skull bones have not yet fused

Septic Shock (Sepsis)—Presence of harmful microorganisms in the blood

Subdural Hemorrhage—Collection of blood in the space between membranes around the brain

Chapter 6

Actigraphy—An actigraph is a small device, similar in size and appearance to a wristwatch, that is worn on the arm or leg to measure frequency and intensity of movement.

Melatonin—A naturally occurring hormone that is important in regulating circadian rhythms and sleep cycles

Polysomnography—A diagnostic test used to record physiological activity during sleep. Usually conducted in a lab during the person's normal sleep schedule, it includes monitoring of brain activity, eye movements, heart rhythms, breathing, and muscle activity.

Sleep Apnea—From the Greek, meaning "without breath," this term refers to disordered sleep where the individual repeatedly stops breathing. It is caused by obstruction of the airway, failure of the brain to signal the diaphragm to breathe, or a combination of the two.

Chapter 7

Antimetabolite—A chemical that inhibits the use of a metabolite. Such chemicals are useful in chemotherapy, as antimetabolites can interrupt the cell division of cancer cells.

B-Cells—Lymphocytes that make antibodies against antigens. They have a memory function so that once they have "learned" a new antigen, they respond much quicker to future occurrences.

Demyelination—Disease or damage to the myelin sheath, a fatty protective coating of neurons that facilitates neuronal transmission, thus causing impairment in cognitive, sensory, and motor domains

Granulocytes—A type of white blood cell produced by bone marrow

Intracranial Calcifications—A condition where calcium and iron deposit on the walls of blood vessels in brain tissue

Intrathecal—Occurring within the spinal column, such as an intrathecal injection that is injected directly into the cerebral-spinal fluid. This is often done so that the medication does not have to pass through the blood-brain barrier.

Leukocyte—A white blood cell. Malignant leukocytes are found in leukemia

Leukoencephalopathy—Brain-based diseases involving white matter (*See* demyelination.)

Lymphocyte—A leukocyte found in the lymphatic system

Monocyte—A type of leukocyte produced by bone marrow that travels the bloodstream and ingests foreign threats

Prophylaxis—Prevention or protection against disease

T-Cells—Lymphocytes that mature in the thymus and are important for immune defense

Chapter 8

Disclosure—The process of telling a child that he or she is HIV positive. Partial disclosure is explaining that the child has an illness but not naming it as HIV. Full disclosure is explaining the entire health condition to the child.

Encephalopathy—Any disease of the brain

Hemoglobin—A part of the red blood cells that binds to oxygen and carries it through the body

Highly Active Antiretroviral Therapy (HAART)—A combination of several medications that interfere with HIV's ability to copy itself and, thus, reduces HIV's concentration in the blood. HAART is often called a drug "cocktail."

Viral Load—The measure of the concentration of HIV RNA or DNA in the child's blood

Chapter 9

Cerebrospinal Fluid (CSF)—A watery fluid, continuously produced and absorbed, that flows in the ventricles (cavities) within the brain and around the surface of the brain and spinal cord

Cranial Nerve Palsy—A paralysis of one or more nerves that pass from the brain to parts of the face and neck

Edema—The swelling of soft tissues because of excess fluid accumulation

Hemiparesis—Muscular weakness or partial paralysis on one side of the body

Meninges—Three layers of tissue that cover the brain and protect the spinal cord

Meningitis—An infection of the fluid of the spinal cord and the fluid that surrounds the brain

Necrosis—The death of living cells or tissues. This can be caused by lack of blood flow.

Nosocomial—Originating or taking place in a hospital or acquired in a hospital, especially in reference to an infection

Parenteral—Taken into the body or administered in a manner other than through the digestive tract, as by intravenous or intramuscular injection

Pathogen—An agent that causes disease

Sensorineural—Hearing loss caused by the damage to the cochlea (inner ear) and/or the hearing nerve

Subarachnoid Space—The middle meningeal layer, filled with spongy blood vessels and canals carrying cerebral spinal fluid, where infections can develop

Chapter 10

Colitis—Inflammation of the colon

Duodenitis—Inflammation of the duodenum

Keratitis—Inflammation of the cornea

Optic Neuritis—Inflammation of the optic nerve that may cause partial or complete loss of vision

Uveitis—Inflammation of the uvea, the middle layer of the eye

Vectored Disease—Disease propagated through intermediate hosts, which carry and deliver parasites to subsequent hosts. Examples include mosquitoes that carry malaria or ticks that carry Lyme disease.

Chapter 11

Body Mass Index (BMI)—BMI is a reliable proxy for body fat that is easily calculated using an individual's height and weight. BMI is used to screen for overweight and obesity because it is inexpensive and easy and correlates well with direct assessments of body fat. When interpreting children's and adolescents' BMI, it is important to take into consideration age and gender. For children and adolescents, BMI is referred to as BMI-for-age.

Body Mass Index (BMI) Percentile—For children and adolescents, BMI-for-age is plotted on sex-specific growth charts to obtain a percentile rank that is used to compare an individual with others who are the same age and gender.

Competitive Foods—Foods or beverages other than those offered at school through the federally reimbursed school meal programs. Competitive foods include food and beverage items sold through à la carte lines, snack bars, student stores, vending machines, and fund-raisers.

"Eating in the Absence of Hunger" (EAH)—A tendency to eat in the presence of palatable foods in the absence of hunger

Energy Balance—A state in which calorie intake equals calorie expenditure, resulting in weight homeostasis (i.e., neither weight gain nor loss)

Obesogenic—Factors that contribute to obesity. *Obesogenic* has been used to describe the environment (i.e., an obesogenic environment), referring to the numerous and ubiquitous elements of our society that interact with each other in complex ways, making it easy to consume and difficult to burn off excess calories.

Weight Status—The Centers for Disease Control and Prevention developed four weight status categories for children and adolescents. A child or adolescent's weight status category depends on his or her BMI-for-age percentile. *Underweight* is defined as less than the 5th percentile; *Healthy Weight* is between the 5th and 85th percentile; *Overweight* is between the 85th and 95th percentile; *Obese* is equal to or greater than the 95th percentile.

Chapter 12

Aggressive-Victim—Individual who is both a perpetrator and a target of aggressive acts. Also known as *bully victim* or *provocative victim*.

Hostile Attribution Bias—Tendency to perceive ambiguous stimuli or acts as having hostile intent

Peer Nominations—Method of assessing social status or behavior in which children are presented with a roster of the names of their classmates and asked to circle the names of children whom they like most and whom they like least.

Relational Aggression—Attempt to harm through influencing an individual's social standing (e.g., by threatening to withdraw friendships, socially excluding, spreading rumors).

Social Aggression—Attempting to harm an individual's self-esteem or social status through influencing relationship patterns, gossiping, or negative facial expressions (e.g., eye rolling). Term is sometimes used interchangeably with *relational aggression.*

Social Information Processing (SIP) Model—Developmental model used to explain child behavior (including aggression) based on series of cognitive steps: (1) encoding of internal and external cues, (2) interpretation of cues, (3) clarification and selection of a goal, (4) response access (i.e., generating alternatives), (5) response decision (i.e., evaluating alternatives), and (6) behavioral enactment

Chapter 13

Traumatic Brain Injury (TBI)—An injury, caused by a blow or jolt to the head or a penetrating head injury, that disrupts the function of the brain. The severity of a TBI may range from mild (i.e., resulting in a brief change in mental status or consciousness) to severe (i.e., resulting in an extended period of coma or amnesia).

Spinal Cord Injury (SCI)—An insult to the spinal cord resulting in a change, either temporary or permanent, in its normal motor, sensory, or autonomic function. An SCI can be classified as either complete (indicated by a total lack of sensory or motor function below the level of injury) or incomplete (the ability of the spinal cord to convey messages to or from the brain is not completely lost).

References

Chapter 1

Brown, M. B., & Bolen, L. M. (2008). The school-based health center as a resource for prevention and health promotion. *Psychology in the Schools, 45,* 28–39.

Clay, D. L., Cortina, S., Harper, D. C., Cocco, K. M., & Drotar, D. (2004). Schoolteachers' experiences with childhood chronic illness. *Children's Health Care, 33,* 227–239.

Cook, B. A., Schaller, K., & Krischer, J. P. (1985). School absences among children with chronic illness. *Journal of School Health, 55,* 265–267.

Kisker, E. E., & Brown, R. S. (1996). Do school-based health centers improve adolescents' access to health care, health status, and risk taking behavior? *Journal of Adolescent Health, 18,* 335–343.

Kyngas, H. (2004). Support network of adolescents with chronic disease: Adolescents' perspective. *Nursing Sciences, 6,* 287–293.

Reeder, G. D., Maccow, G. C., Shaw, S. R., Swerdlik, M. E., Horton, C. B., & Foster, P. (1997). School psychologists and full service schools: Partnerships with medical, mental health, and social services. *School Psychology Review, 26,* 603–621.

Rehabilitation Act of 1973 (Section 504), 29 U.S.C. § 794. Retrieved September 19, 2009, from http://www.ed.gov/policy/rights/reg/ocr/edlite-34cfr104.html

Shaw, S. R. (2003). Professional preparation of pediatric school psychologists for school-based health centers. *Psychology in the Schools, 40,* 321–330.

Shaw, S. R., Kelly, D. P., Joost, J. C., & Parker-Fisher, S. J. (1995). School-linked health services: A renewed call for collaboration between school psychologists and medical professionals. *Psychology in the Schools, 32,* 190–201.

Shaw, S. R., & McCabe, P.C. (2008). Hospital to school transition for children with chronic illness: Meeting the new challenges of an evolving health care system. *Psychology in the Schools, 45,* 74–87.

Stam, H., Hoffman, E. E., Deurloo, J. A., Groothoff, J., & Grootenhuis, M. A. (2006). Young adult patients with a history of pediatric disease: Impact on course of life and transition into adulthood. *Journal of Adolescent Health, 39,* 4–13.

U.S. Green Building Council (USBGC). (2008, August 27). Schools rapidly turning green across America. Retrieved September 19, 2009, from http://www.govtech.com/gt/404167?topic=290183

Chapter 2

American Psychiatric Association (APA). (2000). *Diagnostic and statistical manual for mental disorders* (text revision). Washington, DC: Author.

Benson, J. L., Hughes, C., Helwig, J., & Shapiro, E. S. (2009). Facilitating relationships with pediatricians. *NASP Communiqué, 37,* 1.

Drotar, D. (1995). *Consulting with physicians.* New York: Plenum.

McCabe, P. C., & Sharf, C. (2007). Building stronger, healthier families when a child is chronically ill: A guide for school personnel (Handout). *NASP Communiqué, 36*(1).

National Association of School Psychologists (NASP) Delegate Assembly. (2006, July). *Position statement on interagency collaboration to support the mental health needs of children and families.* Retrieved September 19, 2009, from http://www .nasponline.org/about_nasp/pospaper_iac.aspx

Power, T. J., & Blom-Hoffman, J. (2004). The school as a venue for managing and preventing health problems: Opportunities and challenges. In R. T. Brown (Ed.), *Handbook of pediatric psychology in school settings* (pp. 37–48). Mahwah, NJ: Lawrence Erlbaum.

Segool, N. K., Mathiason, J. B., Majewicz-Hefley, A., & Carlson, J. S. (2009). Enhancing student mental health: Collaboration between medical professionals and school psychologists. *NASP Communiqué, 37,* 1–4.

Shaw, S. R., Clayton, M. C., Dodd, J. L., & Rigby, B. T. (2004). Collaborating with physicians: A guide for school leaders. *Principal Leadership Magazine, 5,* 11–13.

Shaw, S. R., Clayton, M. C., Dodd, J. L., & Rigby, B. T. (2009). Collaborating with physicians: A guide for educators. *NASP Communiqué, 37,* 1–4.

Shaw, S. R., & Woo, A. (2008). Best practices in collaboration with medical professionals. In A. Thomas & J. Grimes (Eds.), *Best practices in school psychology* (Vol. V, pp. 1707–1719). Washington, DC: National Association of School Psychologists.

Chapter 3

Bezáková, N., Damoiseaux, R., Hoes, A. W., Schilder, A., & Rovers, M. M. (2009). Recurrence up to 3.5 years after antibiotic treatment of acute otitis media in very young Dutch children: Survey of trial participants. *BMJ, 339,* b2525–2529.

Butler, C., van der Lindern, M., MacMillian, H., & ver der Wouden, J. (2003). Should children be screened to undergo early treatment for otitis media with effusion? A systematic review of randomized trials. *Child Care Health and Development, 25,* 425–432.

Casselbrant, M. L., Mandel, E. M., Fall, P. A., Rockette, H. E., Kurs-Lasky, M., Bluestone, C. D., et al. (1999). The heritability of otitis media: A twin and triplet study. *JAMA, 282*(22), 2125–2130.

Feldman, H. M., Dollaghan, C. A., Campbell, T. F., Colborn, D. K., Janosky, J., Kurs-Lasky, M., et al. (2003). Parent-reported language skills in relation to otitis media during the first three years of life. *Journal of Speech, Language, & Hearing Research, 46*(2), 273–287.

Golz, A., Netzer, A, Westerman, S. T., Westerman, L. M., Gilbert, D. A., Joachims, H. Z., et al. (2005). Reading performance in children with otitis media. *Archives of Otolaryngology Head and Neck Surgery, 132,* 495–499.

Greiner, A. N. (2006). Allergic rhinitis: Impact of the disease and considerations for management. *The Medical Clinics of North America, 90,* 17–38.

Hall-Stoodley, L. H., Fen, Z. H., Gieseke, A., Nistico, L., Nguyen, D., Hayes, J., et al. (2006). Direct detection of bacterial biofilms on the middle-ear mucosa of children with chronic otitis media. *JAMA, 296*(12), 202–211.

Higson, J., & Haggard, M. (2005). Parent versus professional views of the developmental impact of a multi-faceted condition at school aged: Otitis media with effusions ('glue ear'). *British Journal of Educational Psychology, 75,* 623–643.

James, J. M. (2004). Common respiratory manifestations of food allergy: A critical focus on otitis media. *Current Allergy and Asthma Reports, 4,* 294–301.

Kindig, J. S., & Richards, H. C. (2000). Otitis media: Precursor of delayed reading. *Journal of Pediatric Psychology, 25,* 15–18.

Klausen, O., Moller, P., Holmefjord, A., Reisaeter, S., & Asbojornsen, A. (2000). Lasting effects of otitis media with effusion on language skills and listening performance. *Acta Otolaryngol Supplement, 543,* 73–76.

Kvaerner, K. J., Tambs, K., Harris, J. R., & Magnus, P. (1997). Distribution and heritability of recurrent ear infections. *Annals of Otology, Rhinology, & Laryngology, 106,* 624–632.

Miccio, A., Gallagher, E., Grossman, C., Yont, K., & Vernon-Feagans, L. (2001). Influence of chronic otitis media on phonological acquisition. *Clinical Linguistics & Phonetics, 15,* 47–51.

Nsouli, T. M., Nsouli, S. M., Linde, R. E., O'Mara, F., Scanlon, R. T., & Bellanti, J. A. (1994). Role of food allergy in serous otitis media. *Annals of Allergy, Asthma, & Immunology, 73,* 215–219.

Petinou, K., Schwartz, R., Gravel, J., & Raphael, L. (2001). A preliminary account of phonological and morphological perception in young children with and without otitis media. *International Journal of Language, 36,* 21–42.

Pichichero, M. E. (2000, April 1). Acute otitis media: Part I. Improving diagnostic accuracy. *American Family Physician.* Retrieved September 19, 2009, from http://www.aafp.org/afp/20000401/2051.html

Polka, L., & Rvachew, S. (2005). The impact of otitis media with effusion on infant phonetic perception. *Infancy, 8,* 101–117.

Pshetizky, Y., Naimer, S., & Schvartzman, P. (2003). Acute otitis media—A brief explanation to parents and antibiotic use. *Family Practice, 20,* 417–419.

Reichman, J., & Healey, W. C. (1983). Learning disabilities and conductive hearing loss involving otitis media. *Journal of Learning Disabilities, 16,* 272–278.

Roberts, J., Hunter, L., Gravel, J., Rosenfeld, R., Berman, S., Haggard, M., et al. (2004). Otitis media, hearing loss, and language learning controversies and current research. *Developmental and Behavior Pediatrics, 25,* 110–122.

Secord, G. J., Erickson, M. T., & Bush, J. P. (1988). Neuropsychological sequelae of otitis media in children and adolescents with learning disabilities. *Journal of Pediatric Psychology, 13,* 531–542.

Shriberg, L., Flipsen, P., Kwiatkowski, J., & McSweeny, J. (2003). A diagnostic marker for speech delay associated with otitis media with effusion: The intelligibility-speech gap. *Clinical Linguistics & Phonetics, 17,* 507–528.

Shriberg, L., Friel-Patti, S., Flipsen, P., & Brown, R. (2000). Otitis media, fluctuant hearing loss, and speech-language outcomes: A preliminary structural equation model. *Journal of Speech, Language & Hearing Research, 43,* 100–120.

Williams, R. L., Chalmers, T. C., Stange, K. C., Chalmers, F. T., & Bowlin, S. J. (1993). Use of antibiotics in preventing recurrent acute otitis media and in treating otitis media with effusion: A meta-analytic attempt to resolve the brouhaha. *JAMA, 270,* 1344–1351.

Winskel, H. (2006). The effects of an early history of otitis media on children's language and literacy skill development. *British Journal of Educational Psychology, 76,* 727–744.

Zeisel, S., & Roberts, J. (2003). Otitis media in young children with disabilities. *Infants and Young Children, 16*(2), 106–119.

Chapter 4

American Academy of Pediatrics (AAP). (2008). Recommended immunization schedule for persons aged 0–6 years. Retrieved September 19, 2009, from http://www.cispimmunize.org/IZSchedule_childhood.pdf

Ball, L. K., Ball, R., & Pratt, R. D. (2001). An assessment of thimerosal use in childhood vaccines. *Pediatrics, 107,* 1147–1154.

Bazin, H. (2003). A brief history of the prevention of infectious diseases by immunizations. *Comparative Immunology Microbiology and Infectious Diseases, 26*, 293–308.

Brown, A. (2008). Hot topic: Vaccines and autism. *Parents, 83*(7), 38–39.

Deer, B. (2009, February 8). MMR doctor Andrew Wakefield fixed data on autism. *The Sunday Times*. Retrieved September 19, 2009, from http://www.timesonline.co.uk/tol/life_and_style/health/article5683671.ece

Dinsmoor, R. (1998). The dark side of immunizations. *Science News, 19*(3), 6.

Fombonne, E. (1999). The epidemiology of autism: A review. *Psychological Medicine, 29*, 769–786.

Gellin, B. G., Malbach, E. W., & Marcuse, E. K. (2000). Do parents understand immunizations? A national telephone survey. *Pediatrics, 106*, 1097–1102.

Gruber, C., Nilsson, L., & Bjorksten, B. (2001). Do early childhood immunizations influence the development of atopy and do they cause allergic reaction? *Pediatric Allergy and Immunology, 12*, 296–311.

Halsey, N. A., & Hyman, S. L. (2001). Measles-Mumps-Rubella vaccine and autistic spectrum disorder: Report from the new challenges in childhood immunizations conference convened in Oak Brook, Illinois, June 12–13, 2000. *Pediatrics, 107*, e84.

Health Resources and Services Administration (HRSA). (2008). *National vaccine injury compensation program (VICP)*. Retrieved September 19, 2009. from http://www.hrsa.gov/vaccinecompensation/

Kimmel, S. R. (2003). A mother who refuses to vaccinate her child. *American Family Physician, 67*(3), 651–656.

Lochhead, B. A. (1991). Failure to immunize children under 5 years: A literature review. *Journal of Advanced Nursing, 16*, 130–137.

Maitra, A., Sherriff, A., Griffiths, M., & Henderson, J. (2004). Pertussis vaccination in infancy and asthma or allergy in later childhood: Birth cohort study. *BMJ, 328*, 925–926.

Mathews, T. J., & MacDorman, M. F. (2007). Infant mortality statistics from the 2004 period: Linked birth/infant death data set. *National Vital Statistics Reports, 55*(14), 2007–1120. Available (rev. June 13, 2007) September 19, 2009, at http://www.cdc.gov/nchs/data/nvsr/nvsr55/nvsr55_14.pdf

Nelson, K. B., & Bauman, M. L. (2003). Thimerosal and autism? *Pediatrics, 111*, 674–679.

Novotny, T., Jennings, C. E., Doran, M., March, C. R., Hopkins, R. S., Wassilak, S. G. F., et al. (1988). Measles outbreak in religious groups exempt from immunization laws. *Public Health Reports, 103*, 49–54.

Offit, P. A. (2008). Vaccines and autism revisited—The Hannah Poling case. *The New England Journal of Medicine, 358*, 2089–2091.

Offit, P. A., Quarles, J., Gerber, M. A., Hackett, C. J., Marcuse, E. K., Kollman, T. R., et al. (2002). Addressing parents' concerns: Do multiple vaccines overwhelm or weaken the infant's immune system? *Pediatrics, 109*, 124–129.

Osterling, J., & Dawson, G. (1994). Early recognition of children with autism: A study of first birthday home videotapes. *Journal of Autism and Developmental Disorder, 24*, 247–257.

Peel, M. (2004). Nigerian islamists veto vaccines. *Academic Search Premier, 96*(86), 6–7.

Stern, A. M., & Markel, H. (2005). The history of vaccines and immunization: Familiar pattern, new challenges. *Health Affairs, 24*(3), 611–621.

Sundqwist, M., Trollfors, B., & Taranger, J. (1998). Pertussis in infancy does not increase the risk of asthma. *Pediatrics, 102*, 1496–1497.

Wakefield, A. J., Murch, S. H., Anthony, A., Linnel, J., Casson, D. M., Malik, M., et al. (1998). Ileal-lymphoid-nodular hyperplasia, non-specific colitis, and pervasive developmental disorder in children. *Lancet, 351*, 637–641.

Zent, O., Arras-Reiter, C., Broeker, M., & Hennig, R. (2002). Immediate allergic reactions after vaccinations—A post-marketing surveillance review. *European Journal of Pediatrics, 161*, 21–25.

Chapter 5

American Academy of Pediatrics (AAP) Committee on Child Abuse and Neglect. (2001). Shaken baby syndrome: Rotational cranial injuries—technical report. *Pediatrics, 108*, 206–210.

Brooks, W., & Weathers, L. (2001). Who are the perpetrators and why do they do it? In S. Lazoritz & V. Palusci (Eds.), *The shaken baby syndrome: A multidisciplinary approach* (pp. 1–8). Binghamton, NY: Haworth Maltreatment and Trauma Press.

Butler, G. L. (1995). Shaken baby syndrome. *Journal of Psychosocial Nursing, 33*, 47–50.

Chiocca, E. M. (1995). Shaken baby syndrome: A nursing perspective. *Pediatric Nursing, 21*, 33–38.

Christian, C. W., Block, R., & American Academy of Pediatrics Committee on Child Abuse and Neglect. (2009). Abusive head trauma in infants and children. *Pediatrics, 123*, 1409–1411.

Davies, W., & Garwood, M. (2001). Who are the perpetrators and why do they do it? In S. Lazoritz & V. Palusci (Eds.), *The shaken baby syndrome: A multidisciplinary approach* (pp. 41–54). Binghamton, NY: Haworth Maltreatment and Trauma Press.

Dias, M., Smith, K., deGuehery, K., Mazur, P., Li, V., & Shaffer, M. (2005). Preventing abusive head trauma among infants and young children: A hospital-based, parent education program. *Pediatrics, 115*, e470–e477.

Dorfman, D., & Paradise, J. (1995). Emergency diagnosis and management of physical abuse and neglect of children. *Current Opinion in Pediatric Ophthalmology, 7*, 297–301.

Ennis, E., & Henry, M. (2004). A review of social factors in the investigation and assessment of non-accidental head injury to children. *Pediatric Rehabilitation, 7*, 205–214.

Gedieit, R. (2001). Medical management of the shaken infant. In S. Lazoritz & V. Palusci, (Eds.), *The shaken baby syndrome: A multidisciplinary approach* (pp. 155–171). Binghamton, NY: Haworth Maltreatment and Trauma Press.

Gutierrez, F. L., Clements, P. T., & Averill, J. (2004). Shaken baby syndrome: Assessment, intervention, & prevention. *Journal of Psychosocial Nursing & Mental Health Services, 42*(12), 22–29.

Hennes, H., Kini, N., & Palusci, V. (2001). The epidemiology, clinical characteristics and public health implications of shaken baby syndrome. In S. Lazoritz & V. Palusci (Eds.), *The shaken baby syndrome: A multidisciplinary approach* (pp. 19–40). Binghamton, NY: Haworth Maltreatment and Trauma Press.

Isser, N., & Schwartz, L. (2006). Shaken baby syndrome. *Journal of Psychiatry & Law, 34*, 291–306.

Kapoor, S., Schiffman, J., Tang, R., Kiang, E., Li, H., & Woodward, J. (1997). The significance of white-centered retinal hemorrhages in the shaken baby syndrome. *Pediatric Emergency Care, 13*, 183–185.

Karandikar, S., Coles, L., Jayawant, S., & Kemp, A. (2004). The neurodevelopmental outcome in infants who have sustained a subdural haemorrhage from non-accidental head injury. *Child Abuse Review, 13*, 178–187.

Keenan, H., & Runyan, D. (2001). Shaken baby syndrome: Lethal inflicted traumatic brain injury in young children. *North Carolina Medical Journal, 62*, 345–348.

Kemp, A. M., & Coles, L. (2003). The role of health professionals in preventing non-accidental head injury. *Child Abuse Review, 12*(6), 374–383.

Kivlin, J. (2001). Manifestations of the shaken baby syndrome. *Current Opinion in Ophthalmology, 12*, 158–163.

Kruger, N. (1997). Shaken baby syndrome: Identification and prevention by early childhood educators. *South African Journal of Education, 17*, 107–115.

Lancon, J., Haines, D., & Parent, A. (1998). Anatomy of the shaken baby syndrome. *The Anatomical Record, 253*, 13–18.

McCabe, C., & Donahue, S. (2000). Prognostic indicators for vision and mortality in shaken baby syndrome. *Archives of Ophthalmology, 118*, 373–376.

Miehl, N. (2005). Shaken baby syndrome. *Journal of Forensic Nursing, 1*, 111–117.

Nagler, J. (2002). Child abuse and neglect. *Current Opinion on Pediatrics, 14*, 251–254.

Pantrini, S. (2002). A window of opportunity: Preventing shaken baby syndrome in A&E. *Pediatric Nursing, 14*, 32–34.

Riffenburgh, R., & Sathyavagiswaran, L. (1991a). The eyes of child abuse victims: Autopsy findings. *Journal of Forensic Science, 36*, 741–747.

Riffenburgh, R., & Sathyavagiswaran, L. (1991b). Ocular findings at autopsy of child abuse victims. *Ophthalmology, 98*, 1519–1524.

Showers, J. (2001). Preventing shaken baby syndrome. In S. Lazoritz & V. Palusci (Eds.), *The shaken baby syndrome: A multidisciplinary approach* (pp. 349–366). Binghamton, NY: Haworth Maltreatment and Trauma Press.

State Education Department, University of the State of New York (USNY). (2002). *Traumatic brain injury: A guidebook for educators.* Albany, NY: Author. Originally printed 1995. (ERIC Document Reproduction Service No. ED452619; reprint available September 19, 2009, from http://www.vesid.nysed.gov/specialed/tbi/guidebook.pdf)

Swenson, J., & Levitt, C. (1997). Shaken baby syndrome: Diagnosis and prevention. *Minnesota Medicine, 80*, 41–44.

Togioka, B. M., Arnold, M. A., Bathurst, M. A., Ziegfeld, S. M., Nabaweesi, R., Colombani, P. M., et al. (2009). Retinal hemorrhages and shaken baby syndrome: An evidence-based review. *Journal of Emergency Medicine, 37*, 98–106.

Wheeler, P. (2003). Shaken baby syndrome—An introduction to the literature. *Child Abuse Review, 12*, 401–415.

Wilkinson, W. S., Han, D. P., Rappley, M. D., & Owings, C. L. (1989). Retinal hemorrhage predicts neurologic injury in the shaken baby syndrome. *Archives of Ophthalmology, 107*, 1472–1474.

Chapter 6

American Academy of Sleep Medicine (AASM). (2005). *The international classification of sleep disorders: Diagnostic & coding manual* (2nd ed.). Westchester, IL: Author.

American Psychiatric Association (APA). (2000). *Diagnostic and statistical manual for mental disorders* (text revision). Washington, DC: Author.

Amin, R., & Daniels, S. (2002). Relationship between obesity and sleep-disordered breathing in children: Is it a closed loop? *The Journal of Pediatrics, 140*, 641–643.

Buckhalt, J. A., El-Sheikh, M., Keller, P. S., & Kelly, R. J. (2009). Concurrent and longitudinal relationships between children's sleep and cognitive functioning. *Child Development, 80*, 875–892.

Buckhalt, J. A., Wolfson, A. R., & El-Sheikh, M. (2009). Children's sleep and school psychology practice. *School Psychology Quarterly, 24*, 60–69.

Carskadon, M. A., & Acebo, C. (2002). Regulation of sleepiness in adolescents: Update, insights, and speculation. *Sleep, 25*, 606–614.

Carskadon, M. A., Dement, W. C., Mitler, M. M., Roth, T., Westbrook, P., & Keenan, S. (1986). Guidelines for the multiple sleep latency test (MSLT): A standard measure of sleepiness. *Sleep, 9*, 519–524.

Chervin, R. D., Hedger, K., Dillon, J. E., & Pituch, K. J. (2000). Pediatric sleep questionnaire (PSQ): Validity and reliability of scales for sleep-disordered breathing, snoring, sleepiness, and behavioral problems. *Sleep Medicine, 1*, 21–32.

Cohen-Zion, M., & Ancoli-Israel, S. (2004). Sleep in children with attention-deficit hyperactivity disorder (ADHD): A review of naturalistic and stimulant intervention studies. *Sleep Medicine Reviews, 8*, 379–402.

Cortesi, F., Giannotti, F., & Ottaviano, S. (1999). Sleep problems and daytime behavior in childhood idiopathic epilepsy. *Epilepsia, 40*, 1557–1565.

Dahl, R. E., & Lewin, D. S. (2002). Pathways to adolescent health: Sleep regulation and behavior. *Journal of Adolescent Health, 31*, 175–184.

Desager, K. N., Nelen, V., Weyler, J. J., & De Backer, W. A. (2004). Sleep disturbance and daytime symptoms in wheezing school-aged children. *Journal of Sleep Research, 14*, 77–82.

Drake, C., Nickel, C., Burduvali, E., Roth, T., Jefferson, C., & Badia, P. (2003). The Pediatric Daytime Sleepiness Scale (PDSS): Sleep habits and outcomes in middle-school children. *Sleep, 26*, 455–458.

Halbower, A. C., & Mahone, E. M. (2006). Neuropsychological morbidity linked to childhood sleep-disordered breathing. *Sleep Medicine Reviews, 10*, 97–107.

Ivanenko, A., Crabtree, V. M., & Gozal, D. (2005). Sleep and depression in children and adolescents. *Sleep Medicine Reviews, 9*, 115–129.

Luginbuehl, M. (2003). *Sleep disorders inventory for students.* San Antonio: Pearson.

National Sleep Foundation. (2004). *2004 Sleep in America poll.* Washington DC: Author.

Owens, J. A., & Dalzell, V. (2005). Use of the 'BEARS' sleep screening tool in a pediatric residents' continuity clinic: A pilot study. *Sleep Medicine, 6*, 63–69.

Owens, J. A., Spirito, A., & McGuinn, M. (2000). The Children's Sleep Habits Questionnaire (CSHQ): Psychometric properties of a survey instrument for school-aged children. *Sleep, 23*, 1–9.

Redline, S. S., Tishler, P. V., Schluchter, M., Aylor, J., Clark, K., & Graham, G. (1999). Risk factors for sleep-disordered breathing in children: Associations with obesity, race, and respiratory problems. *American Journal of Respiratory and Critical Care Medicine, 159*, 1527–1532.

Richdale, A., Francis, A., Gavidia-Payne, S., & Cotton, S. (2000). Stress, behaviour, and sleep problems in children with an intellectual disability. *Journal of Intellectual and Developmental Disability, 25*, 147–161.

Sadeh, A. (2007). Consequences of sleep loss or sleep disruption in children. *Sleep Medicine Clinics, 2*, 513–520.

Sadeh, A., Gruber, R., & Raviv, A. (2003). The effect of sleep restriction and extension on school-age children: What a difference an hour makes. *Child Development, 74*, 444–455.

Stores, G., & Wiggs, L. (Eds.). (2001). *Sleep disturbance in children and adolescents with disorders of development: Its significance and management.* Oxford, England: MacKeith.

U.S. Department of Education. (2008). *Mapping America's educational progress 2008.* Retrieved September 19, 2009, from http://www.ed.gov/nclb/accountability/results/progress/nation.pdf

Williams, P. G., Sears, L. L., & Allard, A. (2004). Sleep problems in children with autism. *Journal of Sleep Research, 13*, 265–268.

Wolfson, A. R., & Carskadon, M. A., Acebo, C., Seifer, R., Fallone, G., Labyak, S. E., et al. (2003). Evidence for the validity of a sleep habits survey of adolescents. *Sleep, 26*, 213–216.

Wolfson, A. R., Spaulding, N., Dandrow, C., & Baroni, E. (2007). Middle school start times: The importance of a good night's sleep for young adolescents. *Behavioral Sleep Medicine, 5*, 102–109.

Chapter 7

American Cancer Society. (2009). All about leukemia—Children's. Retrieved September 19, 2009, from http://www.cancer.org

Anderson, V., Smibert, E., Ekert, H., & Godber, T. (1994). Intellectual, educational, and behavioral sequelae after cranial irradiation and chemotherapy. *Archives of Disease in Childhood, 70,* 476–483.

Armstrong, F. D., Blumberg, M. J., & Toledano, S. R. (1999). Neurobehavioral issues in childhood cancer. *School Psychology Review, 28,* 194–1003.

Brouwers, P., & Poplack, D. (1990). Memory and learning sequelae in long-term survivors of acute lymphoblastic leukemia: Association with attention deficits. *The American Journal of Pediatric Hematology/Oncology, 12,* 174–181.

Brown, R. T., & Madan-Swain, A. (1993). Cognitive, neuropsychological, and academic sequelae in children with leukemia. *Journal of Learning Disabilities, 26,* 74–90.

Buizer, A. I., De Sonneville, L. M., Van Den Heuvel-Eibrink, M. M., Njiokikjien, C., & Veerman, A. J. P. (2005). Visuomotor control in survivors of childhood acute lymphoblastic leukemia treated with chemotherapy only. *Journal of the International Neuropsychological Society, 11,* 554–565.

Butler, R. W., Hill, J. M., Steinherz, P. G., Meyers, P. A., & Finlay, J. L. (1994). Neuropsychologic effects of cranial irradiation, intrathecal methotrexate, and systemic methotrexate in childhood cancer. *Journal of Clinical Oncology, 12,* 2621–2629.

Carey, M. E., Haut, M. W., Reminger, S. L., Hutter, J. J., Theilmann, R., & Kaemingk, K. L. (2008). Reduced frontal white matter volume in long-term childhood leukemia survivors: A voxel-based morphometry study. *American Journal of Neuroradiology, 29,* 792–797.

Carey, M. E., Hockenberry, M. J., Moore, I. M., Hutter, J. J., Krull, K. R., Pasvogel, A., et al. (2007). Brief report: Effect of intravenous methotrexate dose and infusion rate on neuropsychological function one year after diagnosis of acute lymphoblastic leukemia. *Journal of Pediatric Psychology, 32,* 189–193 .

Conklin, H. M., Khan, R. B., Reddick, W. E., Helton, S., Brown, R., Howard, S. C., et al. (2007). Acute neurocognitive response to methylphenidate among survivors of childhood cancer: A randomized, double-blind, cross-over trial. *Journal of Pediatric Psychology, 32,* 1127–1139.

Jankovic, M., & Brouwers, P. (1994). Association of 1800 cGy cranial irradiation with intellectual function in children with acute lymphoblastic leukemia. *Lancet, 344,* 224–227.

Lampkin, B., DeLaat, C., & George, B. (1992). Acute and chronic leukemias. In E. R. McAnarney, R. E. Kreite, D. P. Orr, & G. D. Konerci (Eds.), *Textbook of adolescent medicine* (pp. 419–426). Philadelphia: W. B. Saunders.

Leukemia & Lymphoma Society. (2009). *Leukemia facts & statistics.* Retrieved September 19, 2009, from http://www.leukemia-lymphoma.org

Mennes, M., Stiers, P., Vandenbussche, E., Vercruysse, G., Uyttebroeck, A., De Meyer, G., et al. (2005). Attention and information processing in survivors of childhood acute lymphoblastic leukemia treated with chemotherapy only. *Pediatric Blood & Cancer, 44,* 478–486.

Mulhern, R. K., Fairclough, D., & Ochs, J. (1991). A prospective comparison of neuropsychologic performance of children surviving leukemia who received 18-Gy, 24-Gy, or no cranial radiation. *Journal of Clinical Oncology, 9,* 1348–1356.

Picard, E. M., & Rourke, B. P. (1995). Neuropsychological consequences of prophylactic treatment for acute lymphocytic leukemia. In B. P. Rourke (Ed.), *Syndrome of nonverbal learning disabilities: Neurodevelopmental manifestations* (pp. 282–330). New York: Guilford Press.

Précourt, S., Robaey, P., Lamothe, I., Lassonde, M., Sauerwein, H. C., & Moghrabi, A. (2002). Verbal cognitive functioning and learning in girls treated for acute lymphoblastic leukemia by chemotherapy with or without cranial irradiation. *Developmental Neuropsychology, 21,* 173–196.

Robaey, P., Dobkin, P., Leclerc, J., Cyr, F., Sauerwein, C., & Theoret, Y. (2000). A comprehensive model of the development of mental handicap in children treated for acutelymphoblastic leukaemia: A synthesis of the literature. *International Journal of Behavioral Development, 24,* 44–58.

Rodgers, J., Horrocks, J., Britton, P. G., & Kernahan, J. (1999). Attentional ability among survivors of leukemia. *Archives of Disease in Childhood, 80,* 318–323.

Roman, D. D., & Sperduto, P. W. (1995). Neuropsychological effects of cranial radiation: Current knowledge and future directions. *International Journal of Radiation Oncology, Biology, and Physiology, 31,* 983–998.

Schlieper, A. E., Esseltine, D. W., & Tarshis, E. (1989). Cognitive function in long survivors of childhood acute lymphoblastic leukemia. *Pediatric Hematology and Oncology, 6,* 1–9.

Silber, J. H., Radcliffe, J., Peckham, V., Perilongo, G., Kishnani, P., Fridman, M., et al. (1992). Whole-brain irradiation and decline in intelligence: The influence of dose and age on IQ score. *Journal of Clinical Oncology, 10,* 1390–1396.

Van Dongen-Melman, J. E., De Groot, A., Van Dongen, I. J., Verhulst, F. C., & Hahlen, K. (1997). Cranial irradiation is the major cause of learning problems in children treated for leukemia and lymphoma: A comparative study. *Leukemia, 11,* 1197–1200.

Waber, D. P., Tarbell, N. J., Fairclough, D., Almore, K., Castro, R., Isquith, P., et al. (1995). Cognitive sequelae of treatment in childhood acute lymphoblastic leukemia: Cranial radiation requires an accomplice. *Journal of Clinical Oncology, 13,* 2490–2496.

Waber, D. P., Urion, D. K., Tarbell, N. J., Niemeyer, C., Gelber, R., & Sallan, S. E. (1990). Late effects of central nervous system treatment of acute lymphoblastic leukemia in childhood are sex-dependent. *Developmental Medicine and Child Neurology, 32,* 238–248.

Zins, J. E., Ponti, C. R., & Noll, R. B. (1998). Leukemia (childhood). In L. Phelps (Ed.), *Health-related disorders in children and adolescents* (pp. 392–399). Washington, DC: American Psychological Association.

Chapter 8

1997 USPHS/IDSA report on the prevention of opportunistic infections in persons infected with human immunodeficiency virus. (1998). *Pediatrics, 102*(Suppl. 4), 1064–1086.

American Academy of Pediatrics, Committee on Pediatric AIDS. (1999). Disclosure of illness status to children and adolescents with HIV infection. *Pediatrics, 103*(1), 164–166.

American Academy of Pediatrics. (2003). Human immunodeficiency virus infection. In *Red Book: 2003 Report of the Committee on Infectious Diseases* (26th ed.; pp. 360–382). Elk Grove Village, IL: Author.

Antiretroviral therapy and medical management of pediatric HIV infection. (1998). *Pediatrics, 102*(Suppl. 4), 1005–1062.

Bachanas, P. J., Kullgren, K. A., Suzman-Schwartz, K., Lanier, B., McDaniel, J. S., Smith, J., et al. (2001). Predictors of psychological adjustment in school-aged children infected with HIV. *Journal of Pediatric Psychology, 26,* 343–352.

Battles, H. B., & Wiener, L. S. (2002). From adolescence through young adulthood: psychosocial adjustment associated with long-term survival of HIV. *The Journal of Adolescent Health, 30,* 161–168.

Bisiacchi, P. S., Suppeij, A., & Laverda, A. (2000). Neuropsychological evaluation of neurologically asymptomatic HIV-infected children. *Brain Cognition, 43,* 49–52.

Blanchette, N., Smith, M. L., King, S., Fernandes-Penney, A., & Read, S. (2002). Cognitive development in school-age children with vertically transmitted HIV infection. *Developmental Neuropsychology, 21,* 223–241.

Bose, S., Moss, H. A., Brouwers, P., Pizzo, P., & Lorion, R. (1994). Psychological adjustment of human immunodeficiency virus-infected school-age children. *Journal of Developmental & Behavioral Pediatrics, 15,* S26–S33.

Brouwers, P., Wolters, P., & Civitello, L. (1998). Central nervous system manifestations and assessment. In P. A. Pizzo & C. M. Wilfert (Eds.), *Pediatric aids: The challenge of HIV infection in infants, children and adolescents* (3rd ed., pp. 293–305). Baltimore, MD: Lippincott Williams & Wilkins.

Centers for Disease Control and Prevention (CDC). (2007). *HIV/AIDS surveillance report* (Vol. 17). Retrieved September 19, 2009, from http://www.cdc.gov/hiv/topics/surveillance/resources/reports/2005report/pdf/2005Surveillance Report.pdf

Cohen, J., Reddington, C., Jacobs, D., Meade, R., Picard, D., Singleton, K., et al. (1997). School-related issues among HIV-infected children. *Pediatrics, 100*, e8–e13.

Englund, J. A., Baker, C. J., Raskino, C., McKinney, R. E., Lifschitz, M. H., Petrie, B., et al. (1996). Clinical and laboratory characteristics of a large cohort of symptomatic, human immunodeficiency virus-infected infants and children. *Pediatric Infectious Disease Journal, 15*, 1025–1036.

Funck-Brentano, I., Costagliola, D., Seibel, N., Straub, E., Tardieu, M., & Blanche, S. (1997). Patterns of disclosure and perception of human immunodeficiency virus in infected elementary school-age children. *Archives of Pediatric and Adolescent Medicine, 151*, 978–985.

Gerson, A. C., Joyner, M., Fosarelli, P., Butz, A., Wissow, L., Lee, S., et al. (2001). Disclosure of HIV diagnosis to children: When, where, why, and how. *Journal of Pediatric Health Care, 15*, 161–167.

Jeremy, R. J., Kim, S., Nozyce, M., Nachman, S., Mcintosh, K., Pelton, S. I., et al. (2005). Neuropsychological functioning and viral load in stable antiretroviral therapy-experienced HIV-infected children. *Pediatrics, 115*, 380–388.

Lindsey, J. C., Malee, K. M., Brouwers, P., & Hughes, M. D. (2007). Neurodevelopmental functioning in HIV-infected infants and young children before and after the introduction of protease inhibitor-based highly active antiretroviral therapy. *Pediatrics, 119*, E681–E693.

Mellins, C. A., Brackis-Cott, E., Dolezal, C., Richards, A., Nicholas, A., & Abrams, E. (2001). Patterns of HIV status disclosure to perinatally infected HIV-positive children and subsequent mental health outcomes. *Clinical Child Psychology and Psychiatry, 7*, 101–114.

Nassau, J. H, Tien, K., & Fritz, G. K. (2008). Review of the literature: Integrating psychoneuroimmunology into pediatric chronic illness interventions. *Journal of Pediatric Psychology, 33*, 195–207.

Nozyce, M. L., Lee, S. S., Wiznia, A., Nachman, S., Mofenson, M. E., Smith, M. E., et al. (2006). A behavioral and cognitive profile of clinically stable HIV-infected children. *Pediatrics, 117*, 763–770.

Pao, M., Lyon, M., D'Angelo, L. J., Schuman, W. B., Tipnis, T., & Mrazek, D. A. (2000). Psychiatric diagnoses in adolescents seropositive for the human immunodeficiency virus. *Archives of Pediatrics and Adolescent Medicine, 154*, 240–244.

Renwick, R., Goldie, R. S., & King, S. (2007). Children, families, and HIV infection. In I. Brown & M. Percy (Eds.), *A comprehensive guide to intellectual and developmental disabilities* (pp. 269–278). Baltimore, M.D.: Brookes.

Roberts, J. (2000). Paediatric HIV/AIDS: A review of neurological and psychosocial implications of infection. *Canadian Journal of School Psychology, 15*, 19–34.

Rutstein, R., Josephs, J., Guar, A., Flynn, P., Spector, S., & Gebo, K. (2007, February). *Mental health and special education issues in a cohort of HIV-infected children: Results from a multisite survey.* Poster at the 14th Conference on Retroviruses and Opportunistic Infections, Los Angeles, CA.

Shanbhag, M. C., Rutstein, R. M., Zaoutis, T., Zhao, H., Chao, D., & Radcliffe, J. (2005). Neurocognitive functioning in pediatric human immunodeficiency virus infection: Effects of combined therapy. *Archives of Pediatric and Adolescent Medicine, 159*, 651–656.

Smith, R. A., Martin, S. C., & Wolters, P. L. (2004). Pediatric and adolescent HIV/AIDS. In R. T. Brown (Ed.), *Handbook of pediatric psychology in school settings* (pp. 195–220). Mahwah, NJ: Lawrence Erlbaum Associates.

Wachsler-Felder, J. L., & Golden, C. J. (2002). Neuropsychological consequences of HIV in children: A review of current literature. *Clinical Psychology Review, 22*, 441–462.

Watkins, J. M., Cool, V. A., Usner, D., Stehbens, J. A., Nichols, S., Loveland, K. A., et al. (2000). Attention in HIV-infected children: Results from the Hemophilia Growth and Development Study. *Journal of the International Neuropsychological Society, 6*, 443–454.

Wiener, L., Mellins, C. A., Marhefka, S., & Battles, H. B. (2007). Disclosure of an HIV diagnosis to children: History, current research, and future directions. *Journal of Developmental and Behavioral Pediatrics, 28*, 155–166.

Yi, M. S., Mrus, J. M., Wade, T. J., Ho, M. L., Hornung, R. W., Cotton, S., et al. (2006). Religion, spirituality, and depressive symptoms in patients with HIV/AIDS. *Journal of General Internal Medicine, 21*, S21–S27.

Chapter 9

Anderson, V., Anderson, P., Grimwood, K., & Nolan, T. (2004). Cognitive and executive function 12 years after childhood bacterial meningitis: Effect of acute neurologic complications and age of onset. *Journal of Pediatric Psychology, 29*, 67–81.

Anderson, V. A., Bond, L., Catroppa, C., & Grimwood, K. (1997). Childhood bacterial meningitis: Impact of age at illness and acute medical complications on long term outcome. *Journal of the International Neuropsychological Society, 3*, 147–158.

Anderson, V. A., & Taylor, H. G. (2000). Meningitis. In K. O. Yeates, M. D. Ris, & H. G. Taylor (Eds.), *Pediatric neuropsychology: Research, theory, and practice* (pp. 117–148). New York: Guilford Press.

Berg, S., Trollfors, B., Hugosson, S., Fernell, E., & Svensson, E. (2002). Long-term follow-up of children with bacterial meningitis with emphasis on behavioural characteristics. *European Journal of Pediatrics, 161*, 330–336.

Centers for Disease Control and Prevention. (2009). *Meningitis.* Retrieved September 19, 2009, from http://www.cdc.gov/meningitis/index.html

Chavez-Bueno, S., & McCracken, G. H., Jr. (2005). Bactieral meningitis in children. *Pediatric Clinics of North America, 52*, 795–810.

Chinchankar, N., Mane, M., Bhave, S., Bapat, S., Bavdekar, A., Pandat, A., et al. (2002). Diagnosis and outcome of acute bacterial meningitis in early childhood. *Indian Pediatrics, 39*, 914–921.

de Louvois, J., Halket, S., & Harvey, D. (2005). Neonatal meningitis in England and Wales: Sequelae at 5 years of age. *European Journal of Pediatrics, 164*, 730–734.

Grimwood, K. (2001). Legacy of bacterial meningitis in infancy. *BMJ, 323*, 523–524.

Grimwood, K., Anderson, V. A., Bond, L, Catroppa, C., Hore, R. L., Keir, E. H., et al. (1995). Adverse outcomes of bacterial meningitis in school-age survivors. *Pediatrics, 95*, 646–656.

Guerra-Romero, L., Tureen, J., & Tauber, M. (1992). Pathogenesis of central nervous system injury in bacterial meningitis. *Antibiotic Chemotherapy, 45*, 18–29.

Halket, S., de Louvois, J., Holt, D. E., & Harvey, D. (2003). Long term follow up after meningitis in infancy: Behaviour of teenagers. *Archives of Disease in Childhood, 88*, 395–398.

Koomen, I., Grobbee, D. E., Jennekens-Schinkel, A., Roord, J. J., & van Furth, A. M. (2003). Parental perception of educational, behavioural and general health problems in school-age survivors of bacterial meningitis. *Acta Paediatrica, 92*, 177–186.

Koomen, I., Grobbee, D. E., Roord, J. J., Donders, R., Jennekens-Schinkel, A., & van Furth, A. M. (2003). Hearing loss at school age in survivors of bacterial meningitis: Assessment, incidence, and prediction. *Pediatrics, 112,* 1049–1053.

Koomen, I., Raat, H., Jennekens-Schinkel, A., Grobbee, D. E., Roord, J. J., & van Furth, A. M. (2005). Academic and behavioral limitations and health-related quality of life in school-age survivors of bacterial meningitis. *Quality of Life Research, 14,* 1563–1572.

Meningitis in children. (1999). *JAMA, 281,* 1560.

Michael, P. (2002). Preventing and treating meningococcal meningitis. *Medsurg Nursing, 11,* 9–13.

Nau, R., & Bruck, W. (2002). Neuronal injury in bacterial meningitis: Mechanisms and implications for therapy. *Trends in Neurosciences, 25,* 38–45.

Parini, S. (2002). The meningitis mind-bender. *Nursing Management, 33,* 21–25.

Phillips, E. J., & Simor, A. E. (1998). Bacterial meningitis in children and adults: Changes in community-acquired disease may affect patient care. *Postgraduate Medicine, 103*(3), 102–117.

Sáez-Llorens, X., & McCracken, G. H., Jr. (2003). Bacterial meningitis in children. *The Lancet, 361,* 2138–2149.

Scheld, W. M., Koedel, U., Nathan, B., & Pfister, H. W. (2002). Pathophysiology of bacterial meningitis: Mechanism(s) of neuronal injury. *Journal of Infectious Diseases, 186,* S225–S233.

Thompson, M. J., Ninis, N., Perera, R., Mayon-White, R., Phillips, C., Bailey, L., et al. (2006). Clinical recognition of meningococcal disease in children and adolescents. *The Lancet, 367,* 397–403.

Weir, E. (2002). Meningococcal disease: Oh no, not another childhood vaccine. *Canadian Medical Association Journal, 166,* 1064–1066.

Chapter 10

Adams, W. V., Rose, C. D., Eppes, S. C., & Klein, J. D. (1999). Cognitive effects of Lyme disease in children: A 4 year followup study. *Journal of Rheumatology, 26,* 1190–1194.

Americans with Disabilities Act (ADA) of 1990, 42 U.S.C. § 12101 *et seq.* Retrieved September 19, 2009, from http://www.ed.gov/about/offices/list/ocr/docs/hq9805.html

Berenbaum, S. (2004). Lyme disease in children and adolescents: Parenting dilemmas. *Lyme Times, 36,* 16–18.

Betz, C. L. (2001). Use of 504 plans for children and youth with disabilities: Nursing application. *Pediatric Nursing, 27,* 347–352.

Bloom, B. J., Wyckoff, P. M., Meissner, H. C., & Steere, A. C. (1998). Neurocognitive abnormalities in children after classic manifestations of Lyme disease. *Pediatric Infectious Disease Journal, 17,* 189–196.

Boyce, M. H., Gelfman, M. H., & Schwab, N. (2000). School health services after *Cedar Rapids independent school district v. Garret F. Journal of School Nursing, 16,* 54–59.

Bransfield, R. C. (2001, April). *Lyme neuroborreliosis and aggression.* Paper presented at the 14th International Scientific Conference on Lyme Disease and Other Tick-Borne Disorders, Farmington, CT. Retrieved September 19, 2009, from http://actionlyme.50megs.com/neuroborreliosis%20aggression.htm

Bransfield, R. C. (2007). Lyme disease, comorbid tick-borne disease, and neuropsychiatric disorders. *Psychiatric Times, 24,* 59–62.

Bransfield, R. C. (2009). Preventable cases of autism: Relationship between chronic infectious diseases and neurological outcome. *Pediatric Health, 3*(2), 125–140.

Bransfield, R., Brand, S., & Sherr, V. (2001). Treatment of patients with persistent symptoms and a history of Lyme disease. *New England Journal of Medicine, 345,* 1424–1425.

Bransfield, R. C., Wulfman, J. S., Harvey, W. T., & Ysman, A. I. (2008). The association between tick-borne infections, Lyme borreliosis, and autism spectrum disorders. *Medical Hypothesis, 70,* 967–974.

Brown, S. L., Hansen, S. L., Langone, J. J., Lowe, N., & Pressly, N. (1999, Summer). Lyme disease test kits: Potential for misdiagnosis. *FDA Medical Bulletin.* Retrieved September 19, 2009, from http://www.lymecryme.com/USDA_Lyme%20Disease%20Test%20Kits_%20Potential%20for%20Misdiagnosis.pdf

Cavendish, R. (2003). A Lyme disease case study and individualized healthcare plan. *Journal of School Nursing, 19,* 81–88.

Centers for Disease Control and Prevention (CDC). (2007). Lyme disease—United States, 2003–2005. *Morbidity and Mortality Weekly Report (MMWR), 56*(23), 573–576. Retrieved September 19, 2009, from http://www.cdc.gov/mmwr/preview/mmwrhtml/mm5623a1.htm

Centers for Disease Control and Prevention (CDC). (2008). Notice to readers: Final 2007 reports of nationally notifiable infectious diseases. *Morbidity and Mortality Weekly Report (MMWR), 57*(33), 901, 903–913. Retrieved September 19, 2009, from http://www.cdc.gov/mmwr/preview/mmwrhtml/mm5733a6.htm

Chen, J. P. (2008). Lyme carditis: Another diagnostically elusive spirochetal disease. *Scientific Medicine Journal, 101,* 125–126.

Coulter, P., Lema, C., Flayhart, D., Linhardt, A. S., Aucott, J. N., Auwaerter, P. G., et al. (2005). Two-year evaluation of *Borrelia burgdorferi* culture and supplemental tests for definitive diagnosis of Lyme disease. *Journal of Clinical Microbiology, 43,* 5080–5084.

Fallon, B. A., Kochevar, J. M., Gaito, A., & Nields, J. A. (1998). The underdiagnosis of neuropsychiatric Lyme disease in children and adults. *Psychiatric Clinics of North America, 21,* 693–703.

Fried, M. D., Abel, M., Pietrucha, D., Kuo, Y-H., & Bal, A. (1999). The spectrum of gastrointestinal manifestations in children and adolescents with Lyme disease. *Journal of Spirochetal Tick-borne Diseases, 6,* 89–93.

Hajek, T., Paskova, B., Janovska, D., Bahbouh, R., Hajek, P., Libiger, J., et al. (2002). Higher prevalence of antibodies to *Borrelia burgdorferi* in psychiatric patients than in healthy patients. *American Journal of Psychiatry, 159,* 297–301.

Halperin, J. J. (2004). Central nervous system Lyme disease. *Current Infancy Disease Reports, 6,* 298–304.

Healy, T. L. (2000). The impact of Lyme disease on school children. *Journal of School Nursing, 16,* 12–18.

Individuals with Disabilities Education Act (IDEA) of 2004, 20 U.S.C § 1400 *et seq.* Retrieved September 19, 2009, from http://www.wrightslaw.com/idea/law.htm

Klein, J. D., Eppes, S. C., & Hunt, P. (1996). Environmental and life-style risk factors for Lyme disease in children. *Clinical Pediatrics, 35,* 359–363.

Lane, R., Steinlein, D., & Mun, J. (2004). Human behaviors elevating exposure to *Ixodes pacificus* (*Acari: Ixodidae*) nymphs and their associated bacterial zoonotic agents in a hardwood forest. *Journal of Medical Entomology, 41,* 239–248.

McAuliffe, P., Brassard, M. R., & Fallon, B. (2008). Memory and executive functions in adolescents with posttreatment Lyme disease. *Applied Neuropsychology, 15,* 208–219.

Msall, M. E., Avery, R. C., Tremont, M. R., Lima, J. C., Rogers, M. L., & Hogan, D. P. (2003). Functional disability and school activity limitations in 41,300 school-age children: Relationship to medical impairments. *Pediatrics, 111,* 548–553.

Nicolson, G. (2007). Systemic bacterial infections (*Mycoplasma, Clmydia, Borrelia* species) in neurodegenerative (MS, ALS) and neurobehavioral disorders (ASD). *Infectious Disease Newsletter,* 1–9. Available September 19, 2009, at http://www.immed.org/infectious%20disease%20reports/reports/SIBI.Myco.Clam.Borr.NeuroMS.ALS.BhavDis.pdf

Rachman, M., & Garfield, D. A. (1998). Lyme disease and secondary depression: Universal lessons from an uncommon cause. *Psychosomatics, 39,* 301–302.

Rehabilitation Act of 1973 (Section 504), 29 U.S.C. § 794. Retrieved September 19, 2009, from http://www.ed.gov/policy/rights/reg/ocr/edlite-34cfr104.html

Rothermel, H., Hedges, T. R., III, & Steere, A. C. (2001). Optic neuropathy in children with Lyme disease. *Pediatrics, 108,* 477–481.

Rupprecht, T. A., Koedel, U., Fingerle, V., Pfister, H-W. (2008). The pathogenesis of Lyme neuroborreliosis: From infection to inflammation. *Molecular Medicine, 14,* 205–212.

Shaw, S. R. (2005). Cognitive deterioration in children: Review and clinical issues. *NASP Communiqué, 33,* 28–31.

Sherr, V. T. (2004). Human babesiosis—An unrecorded reality: Absence of formal registry undermines its detection, diagnosis and treatment, suggesting need for immediate mandatory reporting. *Medical Hypotheses, 63,* 609–615.

Swanson, S. J., Neitzel, D., Reed, K. D., & Belongia, E. A. (2006). Coinfections acquired from *Ixodes* ticks. *Clinical Microbiology Review, 19,* 708–727.

Tager, F., Fallon, B., Keilp, J., Rissenberg, M., Jones, C., & Liebowitz, M. (2001). A controlled study of cognitive deficits in children with chronic Lyme disease. *Journal of Neuropsychiatry and Clinical Neuroscience, 13,* 500–507.

Vazquez, M., Sparrow, S. S., & Shapiro, E. D. (2003). Long-term neuropsychological and health outcomes of children with facial nerve palsy attributable to Lyme disease. *Pediatrics, 112,* 93–97.

Young, J. D. (1998). Underreporting of Lyme disease. *New England Journal of Medicine, 338,* 1629.

Chapter 11

Adair, L. S. (2008). Child and adolescent obesity: Epidemiology and developmental perspectives. *Physiology & Behavior, 94,* 8–16.

Baker, E. A., Schootman, M., Barnidge, E., & Kelly, C. (2006). The role of race and poverty in access to foods that enable individuals to adhere to dietary guidelines. *Preventing Chronic Disease, 3*(3). Available September 19, 2009, at http://www.cdc.gov/pcd/issues/2006/jul/05_0217.htm

Berry, D., Savoye, M., Melkus, G., & Grey, M. (2007). An intervention for multiethnic obese parents and overweight children. *Applied Nursing Research, 20,* 63–71.

Budd, G. M., & Volpe, S. L. (2006). School-based obesity prevention: Research, challenges, and recommendations. *Journal of School Health, 76,* 485–495.

Campbell, K. J., Crawford, D. A., Salmon, J., Carver, A., Garnett, S. P., & Baur, L. A. (2007). Associations between the home food environment and obesity-promoting eating behaviors in adolescence. *Obesity, 15,* 719–730.

Doak, C. M., Visscher, L. S., Renders, C. M., & Seidell, J. C. (2006). The prevention of overweight and obesity in children and adolescents: A review of interventions and programmes. *Obesity Reviews, 7,* 111–136.

Institute of Medicine (IOM). (2007). *Progress in preventing childhood obesity: How do we measure up?* Washington, DC: National Academies Press.

Jenkins, S., & Horner, S. D. (2005). Barriers that influence eating behaviors in adolescents. *Journal of Pediatric Nursing, 20,* 258–267.

Kral, T. V. E., & Faith, M. S. (2008). Influences on child eating and weight development from a behavioral genetics perspective. *Journal of Pediatric Psychology, 10,* 1–10.

Kubik, M. Y., Story, M., & Davey, C. (2007). Obesity prevention in schools: Current role and future practice of school nurses. *Preventive Medicine, 44,* 504–507.

Mauriello, L. M., Driskell, M. M. H., Sherman, K. J., Johnson, S. S., Prochaska, J. M., & Prochaska, J. O. (2006). Acceptability of a school-based intervention for the prevention of adolescent obesity. *The Journal of School Nursing, 22,* 269–277.

Morland, K., & Filomena, S. (2007). Disparities in the availability of fruits and vegetables between racially segregated urban neighborhoods. *Public Health Nutrition, 10,* 1481–1489.

Neault, N., Cook, J. T., Morris, V., & Frank, D. A. (2005). *The real co$t of a healthy diet: Healthful foods are out of reach for low-income families in Boston, Massachusetts.* Boston: Department of Pediatrics, Boston Medical Center. Retrieved September 19, 2009, from http://www.childrenshealthwatch.org/upload/resource/healthy_diet_8_05.pdf

Ogden, C. L., Carroll, M. D., & Flegal, K. M. (2008). High body mass index for age among US children and adolescents, 2003–2006. *JAMA, 229,* 2401–2405.

Ratey, J. J. (2008). *Spark: The revolutionary new science of exercise and the brain.* New York: Little, Brown.

Riggs, N. R., Kobayakawa Sakuma, K., & Pentz, M. A. (2007). Preventing risk for obesity by promoting self-regulation and decision-making skills: Pilot results from the PATHWAYS to Health Program (PATHWAYS). *Evaluation Review, 31,* 287–310.

Small, L., Anderson, D., & Melnyk, B. M. (2007). Prevention and early treatment of overweight and obesity in young children: A critical review and appraisal of the evidence. *Pediatric Nursing, 33,* 149–162.

Stice, E., Shaw, H., & Marti, N. (2006). A meta-analytic review of obesity prevention programs for children: The skinny on interventions that work. *Psychological Bulletin, 132,* 667–691.

U.S. Department of Health and Human Services (HHS). (2001). *The Surgeon General's call to action to prevent and decrease overweight and obesity 2001.* Rockville, MD: U.S. Department of Health and Human Services, Public Health Service, Office of the Surgeon General. Available September 19, 2009, at http://www.surgeongeneral.gov/topics/obesity/calltoaction/CalltoAction.pdf

Chapter 12

Boxer, P., Edwards-Leeper, L., Goldstein, S. E., Musher-Eizenman, D., & Dubow, E. F. (2003). Exposure to "low level" aggression in school: Associations with aggressive behavior, future expectations, and perceived safety. *Violence and Victims, 18,* 691–705.

Bradshaw, C. P., Sawyer, A. L., & O'Brennan, L. M. (2007). Bullying and peer victimization at school: Perceptual differences between students and school staff. School Psychology Review, 36, 361–382.

Cassidy, T., & Taylor, L. (2005). Coping and psychological distress as a function of the bully victim dichotomy in older children. *Social Psychology of Education, 8,* 249–262.

Chen, X., & French, D. C. (2008). Children's social competence in cultural context. *Annual Review of Psychology, 59,* 591–616.

Cillessen, A. H. N., & Rose, A. J. (2005). Understanding popularity in the peer system. *Current Directions in Psychological Science, 14,* 102–105.

Crick, N. R., & Dodge, K. A. (1994). A review and reformulation of social information-processing mechanisms in children's social adjustment. *Psychological Bulletin, 115,* 74–101.

Crick, N. R., & Dodge, K. A. (1996). Social information-processing mechanisms in reactive and proactive aggression. *Child Development, 67,* 993–1002.

Crick, N. R., & Grotpeter, J. K. (1995). Relational aggression, gender, and social-psychological adjustment. *Child Development, 66,* 710–722.

Crick, N. R., & Grotpeter, J. K. (1996). Children's treatment by peers: Victims of relational and overt aggression. *Development and Psychopathology, 8,* 367–380.

Dodge, K. A. (1980). Social cognition and children's aggressive behavior. *Child Development, 51,* 162–170.

Eslea, M., Menesini, E., Morita, Y., O'Moore, M., Mora-Merchan, M. A., Pereira, B., et al. (2003). Friendship and loneliness among bullies and victims: Data from seven countries. *Aggressive Behavior, 30,* 71–83.

Galen, B. R., & Underwood, M. K. (1997). A developmental investigation of social aggression among children. *Developmental Psychology, 33*, 589–600.

Henry, D. (2001). Classroom context and the development of aggression: The role of normative processes. *Advances in Psychology Research, 6*, 193–227.

Kokkinos, C. M., & Panayiotou, G. (2004). Predicting bullying and victimization among early adolescents: Associations with disruptive behavior disorders. *Aggressive Behavior, 30*, 520–533.

Leff, S. S., Power, T. J., Costigan, T., & Manz, P. H. (2003). Assessing the climate of the playground and lunchroom: Implications for bullying prevention programming. *School Psychology Review, 32*, 418–430.

Mayeux, L., Sandstrom, M. J., & Cillessen, A. H. N. (2008). Is being popular a risky proposition? *Journal of Research on Adolescence, 18*, 49–74.

Paquette, J. A., & Underwood, M. K. (1999). Gender differences in young adolescents' experiences of peer victimization: Social and physical aggression. *Merrill-Palmer Quarterly, 45*, 233–258.

Parkhurst, J. T., & Hopmeyer, A. (1998). Sociometric popularity and peer-perceived popularity: Two distinct dimensions of peer status. *Journal of Early Adolescence, 18*, 125–144.

Pellegrini, A. D., Bartini, M., & Brooks, F. (1999). School bullies, victims, and aggressive victims: Factors relating to group affiliation and victimization in early adolescence. *Journal of Educational Psychology, 91*, 216–224.

Perren, S., & Alsaker, F. D. (2006). Social behavior and peer relationships of victims, bully-victims, and bullies in kindergarten. *Journal of Child Psychology and Psychiatry, 47*, 45–57.

Roberto, A. J., Meyer, G., Boster, F. J., & Roberto, H. L. (2003). Adolescents' decisions about verbal and physical aggression: An application of the theory of reasoned action. *Human Communication Research, 29*, 135–147.

Schwartz, D. (2000). Subtypes of victims and aggressors in children's peer groups. *Journal of Abnormal Child Psychology, 28*, 181–192.

Solberg, M. E., Olweus, D., & Endresen, I. M. (2007). Bullies and victims at school: Are they the same pupils? *British Journal of Educational Psychology, 77*, 441–464.

Thomas, D. E., Bierman, K. L., & the Conduct Problems Prevention Research Group (2006). The impact of classroom aggression on the development of aggressive behavior problems in children. *Development and Psychopathology, 18*, 471–487.

Xu, Y., Farver, J. M., Schwartz, D., & Chang, L. (2003). Identifying aggressive victims in Chinese children's peer groups. *International Journal of Behavioral Development, 27*, 243–252.

Chapter 13

Cassidy, J. D., Carroll, L. J., Peloso, P. M., Borg, J., von Holst, H., Holm, L., et al. (2004). Incidence, risk factors and prevention of mild traumatic brain injury: Results from the WHO Collaborating Centre Task Force on Mild Traumatic Brain Injury. *Journal of Rehabilitation Medicine, S43*, 28–60.

Centers for Disease Control and Prevention (CDC). (2001). School health guidelines to prevent unintentional injuries and violence. *Morbidity and Mortality Weekly Report (MMWR), 50*(RR-22), 1–70.

Centers for Disease Control and Prevention (CDC). (2007a). *Healthy youth! Coordinated school health program.* Retrieved September 19, 2009, from http://www.cdc.gov/HealthyYouth/CSHP

Centers for Disease Control and Prevention (CDC). (2007b). Nonfatal traumatic brain injuries from sports and recreation activities—United States, 2001–2005. *Morbidity and Mortality Weekly Report (MMWR), 56*, 733–737.

Conn, J. M., Annest, J. L., Bossarte, R. M., & Gilchrist, J. (2006). Non-fatal sports and recreational violent injuries among children and teenagers, United States, 2001–2003. *Journal of Science and Medicine in Sport, 9,* 479–489.

Cronin, A. F. (2001). Traumatic brain injury in children: Issues in community function. *American Journal of Occupational Therapy, 55,* 377–384.

Durbin, D. R., Elliott, M. R., & Winston, F. K. (2003). Belt-positioning booster seats and reduction in risk of injury among children in vehicle crashes. *JAMA, 289,* 2835–2840.

Harborview Injury Prevention and Research Center (HIRPC). (2001). *Best practices: Drowning prevention interventions.* Retrieved September 19, 2009, from http://depts.washington.edu/hiprc/practices/topic/drowning/index.html

Jacobsen, P. L. (2003). Safety in numbers: Walkers and bicyclists, safer walking and bicycling. *Injury Prevention, 9,* 205–209.

Klassen, T. P., MacKay, J. M., Moher, D., Walker, A., & Jones, A. L. (2000). Community-based injury prevention interventions. *The Future of Children, 10,* 83–110.

Langlois, J. A., Rutland-Brown, W., & Thomas, K. E. (2004). *Traumatic brain injury in the United States: Emergency department visits, hospitalizations, and deaths.* Atlanta, GA: Centers for Diseases Control and Prevention, National Center of Injury Prevention and Control.

Mayo Clinic. (2007). *Child safety: How to prevent drowning.* Retrieved September 19, 2009, from http://www.mayoclinic.com/health/child-safety/CC00045#

National Center for Injury Prevention and Control (NCIPC). (2006). *Spinal cord injury (SCI): Fact sheet.* Retrieved September 19, 2009, from http://www.cdc.gov/ncipc/factsheets/scifacts.htm

National SafeKids Campaign (NSKC). (2004). *Sports injury fact sheet.* Washington, DC: Author.

National SafeKids Campaign (NSKC). (2005). Follow the leader: Pedestrian safety. In *Safe Kids Week 2005 Checklists* (p. 3). Retrieved September 19, 2009, from http://www.usa.safekids.org/content_documents/SK_Week_2005_checklist.pdf

Rivara, F. P., & Metrik, J. (1998). *Training programs for bicycle safety.* Retrieved September 19, 2009, from http://depts.washington.edu/hiprc/pdf/report.pdf

Safe Kids Worldwide. (2007). *Pedestrian safety.* Washington, DC: Author. Available September 19, 2009, at http://www.usa.safekids.org/content_documents/2007_Fact_Sheet_Pedestrian.doc

Staunton, C., Davidson, C., Kegler, S., Dawson, L., Powell, K., & Dellinger, A. (2005). Critical gaps in child passenger safety practices, surveillance, and legislation: Georgia, 2001. *Pediatrics, 115,* 372–379.

Zaza, S., Sleet, D. A., Shults, R. A., Elder, R. W., Dinh-Zarr, T., Nichols, J. L., et al. (2005). Motor vehicle occupant injury. In S. Zaza, P. A. Briss, & K. W. Harris (Eds.), *The guide to community preventive services: What works to promote health?* (pp. 329–384). New York: Oxford University Press.

Index